Advance Praise for
9 Unconscious Reason
Weight Off ... and What to Do About It!

"There are millions of weight loss tips, diets, fads, free advice, and products out there; and they all serve their purpose. However, none of them target the REAL reason of why we have the body we do. Having worked with Tony Robbins for the past decade, I know that the real secret for lasting change is having the right psychology first and techniques and diet later. *Lose Weight for Life* combines that special key ingredient, plus Janis adds another layer with her ontological background to understand the rituals and beliefs we all need to shift or eliminate in order to create the body we desire and deserve. Anyone who's been unable to keep weight off for good owes it to themselves to pick up this book and get started right away! Life will never be the same!"

—Garrett Binder, Sr. Personal Result Specialist, Robbins Research International

"*Lose Weight for Life* demonstrates real insights into the emotional issues around weight loss and gives keys to make lasting change. By understanding how to shift self-sabotaging patterns, you will be able to get out of your own way and set the stage for successful and lasting weight loss."

—Delicia M. Haynes, MD, Diplomat of the American Board of Family Medicine, Diplomat of the American Board of Obesity Medicine, CEO of Family First Health Center, Founder of Premier Physician Consulting, Creator of "Diabetes Free Naturally" and "Love Yourself to Less" Integrative Medical Weight Loss Method

"Having once struggled with my own eating and now being a Registered Dietitian Nutritionist, I know that healthy living is not always easy. But when 'healthy habits' are performed out of fear in an attempt to 'earn our worth,' true healthy living is not just difficult; it becomes IMPOSSIBLE. Thankfully, there is a better way! In *Lose Weight for Life*,

Janis Pullen really GETS IT. She has walked through the flames for herself and now bares her soul to show the behind-the-scenes work that comes with getting real, choosing love over fear, and claiming a healthy body for life. Diet books are a dime a dozen; Janis' insights are a treasure."

—Darice Doorn, RDN, LD ("Darcy the Dietitian"), www.NorthStarNutrition.net

"I love the book and am recommending it to everyone, not just those who want to lose weight. This is the last weight-loss book you will ever have to read! *Lose Weight for Life* has all the information you need, plus all the information you've never known before, to help you lose weight and create new ways to finally live a fulfilling life. Practice the antidotes to self-sabotage patterns that Janis shares, and I promise you that every area of your life will be transformed!"

—Dr. Gail Feldman, PhD, Clinical Psychologist,
Ontological Coach, Author, and International Speaker

"As a certified hypnotherapist, I am extremely aware of the importance of developing congruence between conscious intention and subconscious programming or conditioning. *Lose Weight for Life* provides an excellent foundation for both understanding and implementing the process to develop this necessary congruence. Anyone serious about losing weight and keeping it off should read this book as a part of a comprehensive weight-loss program."

—Jay Pullen, CMS, CHt

"In my work as a master yoga teacher wellness leader, I work with people every day who are captive to the perplexing challenge of permanent weight loss. Surprisingly, success can be energizing and easy when it's informed by a shift in emotions and mindset—an essential component often missed by regular weight-loss programs, which focus only on the outer work. *Lose Weight for Life* does this and more! Janis is a trusted colleague whose methodology and compassion are stellar. I recommend her book to anyone who wants a transformation from the inside out."

—Laurel Hodory, MS, Experienced Registered Yoga Teacher 500,
Founder of Yoga with Laurel and Wellness-at-Work

"*Lose Weight for Life* beautifully guides the reader to fully understand not only the patterns which may be true for them, but also gives practical guidance for the inner shifts to create personal transformation. This understanding not only impacts weight loss and health but how this may be showing up in becoming our personal best in business, life, relationships, and family.

"As a clinical nurse specialist and business mentor, all too often I have seen that people are given the magic pill, 'Just do this,' but over time, this is not enough to sustain change. Janis clearly and simply addresses the inner shifts required to help the reader to not give up on themselves and to take a holistic approach of diet, exercise, and the mental/emotional components so that the interplay of these components work harmony. And when this happens … so much more is possible for life."

—Mary Schmid, Clinical Nurse Specialist,
Business and Money Breakthrough Mentor, www.YourBrilliantYou.com

"I highly recommend Janis Pullen as a weight-loss expert who knows the lasting changes that can only be made by addressing the root of the problem."

—Ruben Ramirez, DC, Albuquerque, NM. Ramirez Chiropractic:
A Spinal Health and Movement Center

"*Lose Weight for Life* is not the typical weight-loss book in any way. If you want to change your relationship with your weight, Janis' brilliant coaching on this sensitive topic is packed into this insightful book. It is a must-read for everyone who wants a life-changing shift with their body … and with themselves!"

—Kendall SummerHawk, Leading Expert in Women Entrepreneurs and Money

"I had four surgeries in 2010, and in 2011 I decided to join a weight-loss challenge at my gym. If it didn't work, I was ready to second-mortgage my house to pay for lap band or gastric bypass surgery. During the orientation for the challenge, I heard Janis Pullen speak about her program. Her words resonated with me. I KNOW what to eat, I KNOW how to work out, but I don't know WHY I'm eating.

"I really believe that Janis Pullen saved my life! With her guidance I have actually FELT emotions, those things I really haven't felt because I was always eating, and thinking I felt better because of the taste of what I was eating, but feeling guilty for the overeating and the kinds of food I was eating.

"I feel as if a doorway to another timeline has opened, and I stepped in and am now living the life I was meant to. I understand my drive to achieve and my drive to eat and protect myself with food and fat. Janis and her weight-loss program have affected every aspect of my life! My marriage is better (and it was great to begin with), I'm developing and achieving goals in other parts of my life, and I'm making a difference for others!

"I have released over ninety-one pounds to date and continue to work with Janis to release the rest. I believe in this program so much that I joined Janis' Weight Loss Coach Certification and Training Program. I have learned how to start a weight-loss business, including the unconscious sabotage information, marketing, branding, and much more. I feel confident about my new weight-loss coaching business and am grateful to Janis for this certification course! Thank you, Janis!"

—Lisa Orick-Martinez, PhD, Albuquerque, NM.
Ontological Weight Loss Client and Certified Coach

"I knew how to eat right and exercise, but I couldn't figure out why I couldn't do it and lose weight! I was exhausted from trying every diet or exercise program and always starting again with a different program—

tomorrow, next week, or after the holidays. I was so ready to lose weight and get my life back when I met Janis!

"Janis' weight-loss program was exactly what I needed. She understands what is going on beneath the eating, and she truly believes in her clients. I have lost over 40 pounds, and I've kept it off! Her program contains what every diet or exercise program needs in order to work in the long run. I would recommend Janis' programs to anyone who wants to lose weight, find a fulfilling career, or make any changes to better their lives. She has a gift and has given me more than I ever expected!"

—Margie Campbell, Albuquerque, NM.
Ontological Weight Loss Client and Certified Coach

"*Lose Weight for Life* is a powerful tool for anyone who has tried to lose weight and has found that diet and exercise are not enough. When you read it, you will learn what sabotages you from living your best and healthiest life and what you can do to shift those sabotages. Janis helped me break through my sabotages in other areas of my life, and my life is forever changed. I love watching her use these same techniques to help people lose weight, keep it off, and transform their lives. It is a must-have for anyone who wants a fulfilled life."

—Becky J. Benes, Transformational Speaker and Authentic Leadership
Development Coach, www.OnenessOfLife.com

"I've known Janis for several years, both as a client and a colleague. My experience of her coaching, and the inspired, creative, and unique way in which she helps people shed their weight, is uplifting and profound. As you will understand when you read her book, Janis comes to weight loss from the inside out. So in the process of letting go of weight, you will also become aware and let go of unconscious feelings and beliefs that have sabotaged you in other areas of your life.

"The result is that you will not only be physically lighter, but you will be emotionally and energetically lighter as well.

"Because I know that overweight is not just about what food goes into one's mouth, but the beliefs we hold about food, what it triggers when and what we eat, and how those emotions play out in other parts of our lives, I can honestly encourage someone who is struggling with the ups and downs of dieting to read this book: *Lose Weight for Life: 9 Unconscious Reasons You Can't Keep Your Weight Off and What to Do About It.*

"It can change your life!"

—Kailash Sozzani, Coach/Mentor for women entrepreneurs to show up: Authentic – Feminine- Beautiful- Empowered

"Lose Weight for Life: 9 Unconscious Reasons You Can't Keep Your Weight Off… and What to Do About It! provides creative, concise and effective ways to shift your body, and more importantly your heart and mind, to achieve the results you want. Janis' work in this area is truly a fulfillment of her purpose on this planet. Janis' authentic sharing of her own life stories touch your heart and inspire you to stay in action, honor yourself, and celebrate your journey."

—Jamie Sue Johnson, Executive Coach and Motivational Speaker

"I met Janis in 1996 and we became good, supportive friends. I have watched her advance through all of her training and have seen her establish herself as an expert in the health/nutritional field. Her ontological approach to keeping the 'pounds off' does work and is a unique and attainable method for long-term weight loss.

"Now she is sharing her successful methods in her book: *Lose Weight for Life: 9 Unconscious Reasons You Can't Keep the Weight Off and What to Do About It.* I recommend the book and the approach to anyone with weight loss as their goal, as this method does work. It helps others learn how to lose the pounds and how to keep the pounds off."

—Karen Baker Stilson, BA, MA, Retired National Branch Manager and Board Adviser, Certified Wholistic Kinesiologist, Health Coach/Consultant

"To my colleague and friend Janis Pullen: Thank you for your wisdom, coaching, love, and friendship. Your book, *Lose Weight for Life*, is a godsend. I wish I'd had this information when I was working as a wellness coach for a healthcare organization. I could have helped my clients to lasting weight loss so much more had I known about 'Protective Default Mechanism' patterns. And I would have felt greater fulfillment, as I would have been providing better value because my clients would have gotten lasting results.

"Your book needs to be out in the world in a big way, and in every corporate wellness program, because ALL of them will FAIL because they only have 'two legs of the weight loss stool!'"

—Quenby Rubin-Sprague, MHROD, RDN, Corporate Healthcare Leadership Development Specialist, www.linkedin.com/in/quenbyrubinsprague/

"I am so delighted to recommend this book! *Lose Weight for Life* is a game changer in the field of health, wellness, and personal development. Every health practitioner, nutritionist, weight-loss-program provider, and personal trainer needs a copy of this book and should recommend it for their clients. Not only will it help your clients get results, it can also truly help make you a more effective, empathetic, and informed practitioner. I am certainly recommending this book and Janis' work to my clients!

"I have known Janis since 2011 as a friend and colleague through our International Coaching community, IAWC. I know from our conversations, from working with Janis, and from seeing her work with others, that Janis Pullen is the Real Deal when it comes to transforming the unconscious, hidden patterns that prevent most people who struggle with weight and weight-related issues, from returning to a natural state of self-respect, self-love, and empowered self-care principles. She has walked this path herself, and has helped others to do the same by creating a system of inquiry, a loving and strong presence, and a coaching methodology that is magnificent to witness.

"A state of balance and harmony with the body are not just for some 'lucky' people. They are part of the natural state of being human, and everyone who is currently suffering the sadness of not being able to feel that harmony deserves to have the gift of Janis' unique teachings, experience, powerful coaching, humour, warmth, and grace."

—Sue Tsigaros, Mastery Coach, Speaker, and Facilitator, Director of Iris Group Pty Ltd. Sydney, NSW, Australia

"I really loved to read this book! It is very good and full of wisdom and great personal examples, and will be a great help to many people around the globe. Janis Pullen has influenced the lives of many people who struggled with losing weight. In *Lose Weight for Life*, she shares her unique wisdom that applies to much more than just losing weight. The insights in this book can be used for all forms of addictive and compulsive behavior. They will enlighten you and reinforce your understanding of how to master your body, work, and happiness in life."

—Dr. Ellen de Lange-Ros, business coach in The Netherlands (Europe)

"Written by a true expert, *Lose Weight for Life* reads like a compelling story, a wise teaching, a powerful lesson, and a work of the Soul. It's an insightful journey through the multifaceted realm of weight loss. Janis Pullen does a remarkable job of taking you straight to the cause of the effects showing up as excess weight. Her journey and expertise lend to her command of this topic and how it connects to money, intimacy, emotions, and purpose. This book is a must-read for everyone on the journey of self-love, weight loss, and those in the business of helping others."

—Stephanie Trager, Esq., Success Coach and Business Strategist

"Janis Pullen is one of the fiercest and most 'heartful' people I have ever met. I had the good fortune to train her as an ontological coach ten years ago. She is a force of love to be reckoned with. She is full of the opportunity of life not only for herself, but for you as well. She has been to the mountaintop and back, and she will guide you to your personal summit as well. What Janis has written, what she has discovered about being healthy, and what she is sharing in the book *Lose Weight for Life* are simply amazing! Her nine reasons you can't get to your healthy lifestyle FOR LIFE are right on. What a gift! I love her, and I know you will too. Buy it, read it, and apply what you learn TODAY."

—Hans Phillips, Owner of Ontoco Inc., Executive Performance Consultant, Co-Founder of Accomplishment Coaching Leadership and Training Program

Lose Weight for Life

Nine Unconscious Reasons You Can't Keep
Your Weight Off … and What to Do About It!

By *Janis Charlton Pullen*

**Creator of Ontological Weight Loss (O.W.L.):
Your Once-in-a-Lifetime Solution**

Dedication

I dedicate this book to my certified weight-loss coaches, my weight-loss clients, and my executive and entrepreneurial clients, whose courage and tenacity have contributed to creating healthy and fulfilling lives for themselves. All of you have given me the precious gifts of inspiration, validation, fulfillment, growth, insight, love, encouragement, and purpose. I am honored in receiving your trust, supporting your breakthroughs, assisting your transformations, and celebrating your victories.

Acknowledgments

I am deeply grateful for all the love, inspiration, and support I receive in my life from so many. I especially want to thank the following people:

- My husband Jay, who consistently models unconditional love for all humankind. He views people and circumstances through the lenses of compassion and understanding, always supporting my visions and dreams.
- My sister Phyllis, who sees me as my highest and best. She believes in me when I cannot believe in myself. She is my role model for generosity, integrity, thoughtfulness, and commitment.
- My daughter Mindy and my granddaughters, Kaylee and Tya, who inspire me to be my best self, share my wisdom, and provide opportunities for healing—theirs and mine.
- My dear friend of decades, Becky Benes, who knows me better than I know myself. Becky has been an inspiration, a coaching client, a valuable referral provider, a colleague, and a staunch supporter of my coaching skills, insights, and intuition.
- Mary Kay Ash, who was my first business mentor. She celebrated the gifts and talents of women entrepreneurs and believed in balancing priorities of faith, family, and work for ultimate success.
- Hans Phillips, mentor and co-founder of Accomplishment Coaching Training Program, who taught me how to love people until they could love themselves.
- Kendall SummerHawk, mentor and premier trainer for women's business coaching, for her tutoring and role modeling of grace and ease in business. In working with Kendall and her husband, coach Richard Shapiro, I learned that I don't have to be a young, energetic male to be successful. Instead, I can be authentically Janis, integrating body, mind, heart, and spirit in business.
- I have been blessed with several other coaches and mentors through the years. All were perfect for my needs at the time and taught me

much. I acknowledge them all, especially Jamie Sue Johnson, who inspired the subtitle of my program: "Your Once-in-a-Lifetime Solution." Jamie Sue is the Queen of Possibility, teaching me that everything is possible when your heart and intentions are in alignment.

- Carole Hyder, colleague and friend, for her support in launching my first Coach Certification and Training Program in 2013. She tirelessly provided valuable marketing feedback along with her consistent encouragement to release my "baby" to the world.

- Our 2014 Mastery Sisters provided brilliant coaching, expertise, experience, suggestions, ideas, and countless other means of support as I launched my first Coach Certification and Training Program. I list them here as a tribute to their contribution to my professional and personal growth and to the legacy of O.W.L.: Andrea Carter, Dinah Snow Pollard, Ellen de Lange-Ros, Julia M. Felton, Karla Sanchez-Pacheco, Marcelle della Faille, Mary Schmid, Meriflor Toneatto, Nafissa Shireen, Quenby Rubin-Sprague, Ruth Klein, and Sue Tsigaros.

- Shannon Kuykendall, my Virtual Assistant, who brilliantly supported me technically so that I could take my business out to the world. Shannon has provided so much more than technical services. She has contributed loving and patient support, brainstorming, and assistance with each stage of rebranding when it was time for a business reinvention.

- Bethany Kelly has helped me become victorious through my journey of writing and publishing a book. Her knowledge and expertise in publishing are embellished with her ontological coach training, so that she brings acceptance, compassion, and wisdom each step of the way.

- Colleen Fiser's brilliance in project management, marketing strategy, and marketing implementation freed up my time and energy so I could focus on what I love doing most: coaching my clients.

- To all the people who have supported and loved me through my journey, whether listed here or not, I am eternally grateful for having you in my life.

Contents

Preface

I have struggled and suffered with both anorexia and obesity since I was a teenager. In the process of losing and gaining weight, I researched and tried almost every diet known to mankind! I have read hundreds of weight-loss books and articles. I have watched and listened to countless videos and audios on the subject. But even more importantly, I have experienced the suffering and struggling firsthand that overweight people endure, and I have experienced the roller coaster of hope, followed by discouragement and resignation, followed by hope, and so on. I wish someone had written this book when I was searching for answers!

As an experienced certified ontological and facilitative life and business coach, I have continually observed, studied, and learned why people behave the way that they do. I have supported a multitude of clients in getting out of their own way by first uncovering their automatic and predictable sabotage patterns and then replacing those patterns with empowering and supportive behavior in all areas of their lives.

Studies show that most people who lose weight will gain it back and will usually regain more than they lost. Why is this? Because most weight-loss and fitness programs concentrate on only two legs of the weight-loss tripod: diet and exercise. Yet we know that the third leg of the tripod, the mental/emotional/psychological component also known as ontology, must be addressed in order to solve the underlying problem—the REAL reasons we are overweight, not the superficial reasons of improper diet and exercise.

I have identified the nine sabotage patterns which must be shifted in order for permanent weight loss to be possible. In my decades of working with overweight people, results prove that those who distinguish and understand these sabotaging patterns and who also take action to replace them with empowering patterns are those who drop their weight and keep it off forever.

My intent is to provide my clients the support for which I always yearned. Our mission for Ontological Wealth, Weight, and Leadership (O.W.W.L.) is to provide a once-in-a-lifetime solution—a program for people worldwide who have struggled and suffered with weight issues, so that they can live their lives with exponentially expanded joy, freedom, and peace.

To carry out our mission, I created programs and informational products which address the holistic (whole self) components of weight loss, including coaching from both ontological (mental/psychological/emotional) and facilitative (plan/action) coaching arenas. I train coaches, health-minded companies, and weight-loss professionals worldwide in my unique methodology so that they may build highly successful businesses, grow themselves to be "ultimate" wellness coaches, and teach their clients to love and respect themselves while dropping weight permanently and living the life of their dreams.

Introduction

The Eternal Merry-go-round

*H*ave you been unable to maintain your desired weight? Which of these are familiar?

- Have you lost excess weight and then gained it back, perhaps with extra pounds?
- Have you done well for a while but then cannot shed those last few pounds?
- Have you been stuck or kept gaining, not able to drop the pounds permanently?
- Have you called yourself unflattering, ugly, self-deprecating names?
- Are you embarrassed or uncomfortable with your body?
- Is getting dressed a chore rather than fun?
- Have you binged and then starved yourself to compensate?
- Do you have a love-hate relationship with food?
- Have you lost weight for a special event, such as a wedding or reunion, but can't keep it off?
- Have you have tried everything without lasting success?

If you're like most chronically overweight people, you either know about or have tried all kinds of diets and weight-loss programs. These programs all usually work when we stick to them. So with inspiration, hope, and high expectations we make a New Year's resolution or start next Monday or get the high school reunion invitation or have a bad doctor report ... or whatever.

So we lose the weight, feel and look great for a while, and then slowly put the pounds back on, often gaining even more than we originally lost. Maybe we regain it quickly, such as when I took off ten pounds in three weeks with the Colonel Sanders diet and then put it right back on when I polished off the whole pan of my mother-in-law's caramel pecan cinnamon rolls in one day! Maybe we never seem to get any or all of the weight off in the first place.

We become discouraged, resigned, or resentful. We say to ourselves, "I don't have enough discipline." Or we say, "This diet doesn't work." Or we say, "I hate to exercise." Or we say, "I'm too busy to cook." Or we say, "Healthy food is too expensive." Or we say, "My family doesn't want to eat what I'm supposed to eat." We make one excuse after another when we are in the mindset of resignation.

Then something happens, such as that doctor report or that New Year's resolution, and we decide to try again. We go around and around, up and down, over and over again, never making peace with ourselves, with our bodies, and with our food. We are either gaining weight or we are losing it. We are on a merry-go-round carousel, and we can't seem to make it stop.

Jumping Off the Carousel

While this merry-go-round ride is exciting or perhaps entertaining in the beginning, especially when we are in the weight-loss stage or immediately following when we are thrilled to resume eating for pleasure, the ride eventually becomes old and depressing. We can't keep the weight off. We lose self-esteem and confidence. Our resolve turns into resignation. We feel the highs with our perceived success, followed by devastation, self-criticism, and remorse with our perceived failure. We want off this ride.

But if we don't know how to stop the machine, which has surely by now become a predictable pattern, our alternative is to jump off while it's moving. How would that be for you? Do you think you can jump off a spinning carousel? Are you scared? Will you get hurt? Are you afraid of the unknown? Will someone catch you? Do you *even know* *why* the ride never stops or what you *would do after* you did manage to jump? Unless we distinguish the core, root causes of our patterns, they will not change. Fortunately, it's simpler than you might believe to trade in this ride for a new, empowered, rewarding one that gives you a body you love and the peace of mind you crave!

Safe Landing

As a mastery life coach, expert on weight loss, and recovering food addict, I know this merry-go-round ride, and I am honored to share the insights and tools you need to jump off your merry-go-round safely and to move into a powerful and fulfilling "What's Next" stage.

I have identified nine unconscious sabotage patterns that keep us fat, the awareness of which enables us to shift our thinking and release the weight once and for all.

In this book, you will uncover the real, authentic self, the one you knew you could be—fit, healthy, and empowered. You will learn to love yourself and your body. You will discover ways to improve your relationships with yourself, food, others, circumstances, and your life ... forever!

Bottom Line

Simply stated, this book will save your life, provided that, first, you are willing to explore your inner world—"inner space" (vs. "outer space," where many of us would rather focus). Second, you must be willing to follow simple instructions. Keeping weight off forever is an inside job. It isn't always easy, but it is simple. It requires some courage, some willingness, and some practice.

Carline, one of my weight-loss clients, exclaimed to me in the beginning of her program, "Janis, this is too hard!" During her program, she learned it is not hard, merely new and different. When Carline followed the simple, step-by-step methodology, she realized that the program was not difficult and was only a matter of shifting her perspective. (Client names have been changed for confidentiality.)

Through experience in my own weight-loss journey and also through coaching clients, I realize that weight loss is really an inside job. The fat on your body is just the outer symptom, just as compulsive spending, drinking, shopping, or other behaviors are outer symptoms.

Why take the time and effort to do the inner work? Coupled with decreasing risk of heart disease, diabetes, cancer, arthritis, sleep apnea, immobility, joint pain, depression, and a host of other physical results of being overweight, you will get your life back. Your embarrassment and discouragement will evaporate. You will love getting dressed every day. You will enjoy intimate relationships more. You will feel comfortable in your own skin. You will have more energy and vitality. You will be proud of yourself. You will love yourself. I imagine you may have your own additional reasons and benefits in mind. Suffice it to say this: You will get to play on all the rides in this amazing amusement park called your life. That's why it's worth the time and effort!

The good news is that everyone can succeed. We can stop the struggling and learn to love ourselves at a deeper level than ever before. Our experience of life can be one of peace, joy, empowerment, and free flow. What would that be worth to you? Is it worth taking the time for yourself to read this book and create a new body and a new perspective on weight loss?

Welcome to the world of discovery! If you are frustrated, resigned, ashamed, or hopeless, then this book is the right one for you; and this is the right time for you to read it. Whether or not you are working on another weight-loss program, this book is critical in order to succeed.

In this book, you will discover the nine, usually unconscious, reasons you can't maintain your weight permanently and what to do about it. You will also learn how those reasons are automatic defaults for you and how they affect your diet and exercise efforts, despite your strongest intentions. You will learn why willpower has nothing to do with permanent weight loss and maintenance. You will read success stories of actual clients who have taken this journey before you.

By reading this book, you will open a new door and embark on a new path in your weight-loss journey. This path leads to a body you adore, enhanced health and well-being, vitality, connection, and balance. Did I mention self-love and empowerment? Thank you for taking a bold step, or perhaps only a curious step so far, that could transform your life.

I have excerpted information from my various programs for you in this book so that you may begin your journey to permanent weight loss and peace, including action steps to take immediately. Prepare to embark upon the journey of your life with my proven and unique signature methodology.

When you do this work, you will discover secrets about yourself you never knew. You will learn new insights, tools, and strategies to drop your weight. You will free up your emotional and mental blocks. You will learn to integrate your body, mind, heart, and spirit and will learn to love yourself deeply. You will transform your relationship and connection with yourself, others, food, spirit, and life. If you will follow instructions, you too can be fit, fabulous, and fat-free forever through the program. You will learn the nine unconscious sabotaging patterns that keep you fat and the shifts you can make to ensure that you are never fat again. You will also read real stories of clients (and my own story) who have struggled and triumphed, just as you can. You can "Lose Weight for Life!"

If you find yourself slipping back or procrastinating, don't worry! If you have any blocks or resistance in implementing the material, don't criticize yourself! Just forgive yourself and start again. If the resistance or procrastination persists, you may choose to work with me or with one of our other coaches. Remember, just as in any self-help book, people often need an unbiased coach or mentor supporting them with compassionate objectivity and being a fierce advocate as they work through the blocks. Especially in weight loss, a coach can help you identify unconscious sabotages and receive the support, accountability, and encouragement you need to succeed in your journey. When you do want additional support, please refer to the Conclusion and Resources chapter for several ways to take the next step.

Thank you for your commitment to a better life and a healthier body.

How to Use This Book

I wrote *Lose Weight for Life* as support for people who struggle and suffer with excess weight and for the coaches who support them. To get the most value from this book, I recommend that you first read it cover to cover as you would read a novel. Then review each chapter in the order in which they resonate with you, and practice the suggested action steps. As you learn to identify and distinguish how the sabotage patterns show up in your life and as you learn how to practice shifting and integrating the corresponding empowerment patterns, you will see your excess weight melt away, while you transform your relationships to food, exercise, circumstances, others, and yourself. You may also wish to use our companion *Lose Weight for Life Workbook* for additional practice areas.

Welcome to the Beginning!

Again, congratulations on taking this journey with me! I wish you happy exploration and happy travels. Thank you again for your commitment to yourself and to creating a life and a body that you love. Thank you for being my partner as we take the steps together. This program works if you work it ... forever. Welcome to my world of weight-loss success! If you are reading this, then you are ready. Let's get started together right now!

The beginning is vague, confusing, and chaotic for people.
Welcome to the beginning!
—Hans Phillips

My Story

We begin with my story and why I am passionate about teaching people to lose weight and keep it off. I have struggled with weight since I was a child. I remember at an early age asking to be excused from the Thanksgiving dinner table at my grandmother's home. Everyone gasped and asked what was wrong; I still had food on my plate. Our family belief that something was wrong if you didn't finish your meal transferred to me in that very moment.

I was taught that I must eat everything on my plate because the children in China were starving. My dad's words ring as loudly now as they did decades ago: "Take all you want, but eat all you take." Of course, when you are serving yourself, you think you're hungrier than you are, so it's easy to take too much. But you still had to eat it all; our family was a collective member of the clean plate club. The habits were being formed early about not wasting food. I never considered until many years later that, when I ate everything on my plate instead of paying attention to my stomach, I was treating my body as a substitute garbage disposal.

The habits were soon embellished with emotional components of eating. My parents divorced when I was six. I remember thinking, "Daddy left because I was not a good enough little girl." Then my mother died suddenly four months later in December, just before my seventh birthday and Christmas. My young interpretation created the belief that I was not good enough and that I was not lovable. Little did I understand that my mother was bipolar, and that none of this was about me. The same year, in the middle of first grade, my beloved teacher died of cancer. I didn't understand why people I loved left. Shy, lonely, and frightened, my little sister and I went to live with our paternal grandparents, while my father traveled and worked long hours to build his insurance company.

Our grandparents lived quietly and orderly. That's when I learned that "Children should be seen and not heard." I have no memories of sadness, grief, anger, fun, or laughter that year. I learned to suppress my emotions and needs. To make matters worse, my father remarried the following year, and the wicked stepmother syndrome began. She was insecure, jealous, and later became addicted to prescription drugs. She verbally and emotionally abused me, thus solidifying my mindset of being unlovable and not good enough, in fact, worthless. Feeling worthless and unlovable are terrifying ways for anyone, especially a young child, to view herself. So I learned that food could numb and comfort the hole in my heart. I began the road of emotional eating and body image problems as I developed a love-hate relationship with food … and myself.

I also learned as a child that food equals love. Both of my grandmothers were excellent cooks, so when my sister and I visited either of them, I knew they loved us when they prepared our favorite meals. To this day, a homemade lemon meringue pie evokes feelings of love and acceptance.

Fast forward to teen age and early adulthood. Twiggy, the British teenage model, actress, singer, and one of the world's first supermodels, set the standard of beauty for girls during the mid-1960s with her skinny, boy-shaped figure from which her nickname was derived. Other models of that time, such as the "Ultimate '60s It Girl," Penelope Tree, showcased the look that we now call anorexic—thin bodies, sunken cheeks, and eyes like saucers. The curvy and sometimes voluptuous actresses of the 1950s and early 1960s, including Marilyn Monroe and Brigitte Bardot, were no longer role models, especially for girls my age.

With an active lifestyle, my body was fit and toned, not fat. However, I was shapely, with curves, nothing like Twiggy or Penelope. So, from the familiar interpretation of "I'm not good enough," I decided that I WAS too fat and began to crash diet. I tried every diet known to mankind: diet colas as a meal substitute, the grapefruit diet, the cabbage soup diet, diet chocolate squares called Ayds Reducing Candy, meal replacement shakes. Starving and bingeing gave way through the years to no fat, high-carb, low-carb, vegetarian, Atkins, Weight Watchers, Jenny Craig, Nutrisystem, and fasting ... to name a few! I turned into a world expert in weight loss, from my extensive reading and research to my years of experience—my own and others. But something was still missing. For example, for my 20th birthday, I decided to lose 10 pounds in three weeks by eating only Colonel Sanders Kentucky Fried Chicken and cole slaw. It worked, and I was so pleased with myself! The next day I devoured the pan of homemade caramel pecan cinnamon rolls that my mother-in-law baked from scratch, just for me. (Here was another confirmation that food equals love.) Shizzam! I regained all the weight I had lost. Yes, something was still missing in my ability to keep the weight off.

How we do one thing is how we do anything. My belief that I was "unlovable and not good enough" extended through all areas of my life. To further illustrate, the "beautiful" girls at that time had long, straight hair. I hated my naturally curly hair and tried in vain to straighten it, including sleeping all night on curlers made of empty orange juice cans and ironing my hair on the ironing board—until I got caught. (This was a time before blow dryers, electric curlers, or chemical straightening products.) My hair was never straight enough, because a little humidity frizzed it up like a Brillo scouring pad, thus confirming I was "not good enough." Yes, I know this is faulty thinking, but I am being transparent here to shed light on what I thought of myself in those days.

In the career arena, I earned bachelor's and master's degrees, became a certified public accountant in two states, and became a Mary Kay Cosmetics Pink Cadillac Director, later realizing that I had achieved these distinctions to prove to myself and others that I was good enough; I was a perfectionist and a workaholic.

Considering the bad habits, the emotional eating, and the striving to change my body type, it's no surprise that my cycle of gaining and losing weight messed up my metabolism. Between binges, my body thought I was starving, so it became harder and harder to drop the pounds. As I got closer to menopause, my weight would go up and down, but with each cycle the gains were higher and the losses were not as low.

Over the course of 20 years my weight spanned a low of 110 pounds to a high of almost 200 pounds. Both extremes of this 90-pound spread (pun intended) were unhealthy; I am five feet five inches tall with a normal bone structure. One time when I was so proud of myself for losing even more weight, co-workers convinced our receptionist to ask me if I was seriously ill. I couldn't understand their concern for my health, since I still thought I was fat, based on the media glorification of Twiggy, et al. However, it was all too true that when I was skinny, my bones hurt when I was lying in bed or sitting in a hard chair. And I still didn't like myself or my body any better when I was thin.

On the other end of the spectrum, when I really was fat at the high end of my weight gains, I despised myself and my body. I felt ugly and uncomfortable in my clothes. I isolated myself socially, emotionally, and physically due to embarrassment and shame. I lacked energy and vitality. My blood pressure was alarmingly high, and I was prediabetic.

The final straw to this struggling and suffering pattern of being anorexic and obese occurred during a ballroom dance performance in front of 300 people when the zipper on my costume broke, exposing my body's rolls of fat. I had not realized how much weight I had gained since the previous competition when I last wore the costume. I was humiliated and ashamed. I silently declared that something HAD to change.

Desperate for relief, I joined Compulsive Eaters Anonymous, a 12-step program similar to Overeaters Anonymous with the addition of a food plan. This was my first experience with doing inner work—the emotional/psychological/spiritual components, rather than only the physical ones, which addressed only diet and exercise. I released 60 pounds to a healthy 140, and I never became anorexic again. I subsequently engaged in personal development work of many descriptions, including a rigorous coaches' training program specializing in the transformation of human beings. I learned how to transform myself and my own life; I began learning to like myself.

What has happened since then? I've kept my weight stable since the 1990s. I now have a healthy relationship with food. I've learned to love and appreciate myself and my life. I made friends and, therefore, peace with my body, including allowing my natural curl to have its way. (Better late than never!) I've learned to identify and fulfill my needs. I am authentic with my feelings and am not afraid to feel them or to express them. I am aligned with myself inside and out. I am living a life with purpose and joy. I began a new career as a life coach to help others to do the same. I created and teach the Ontological Wealth, Weight, and Leadership programs and certification programs to help others do the same.

No Time Or Money?

I used to say that if I were retired and had more time, I would work out every day. Then I noticed when I was on holiday and *did* have the time, I still did not use my time to work out. I also have said that if I had more money, I would hire a personal trainer to keep me accountable, and I would hire a personal chef to shop for organic, healthy food and to prepare all my meals. Then I observed the journeys of Oprah Winfrey, Kirstie Alley, and Wynonna Judd, who had money, hired chefs, and worked out with personal trainers. To my knowledge, all three remain overweight.

My "reasons" were really excuses. The mindset of not enough time or money shows up in everything we do in life, not just weight loss. How we do one thing is how we do everything. Have you ever said, for example, "I would love to take a vacation, but I don't have enough money"? Or have you ever said, "I would love to spend more time by myself, but my schedule is too full"?

What's up with this "lack mentality" regarding time and money? Why isn't anything enough? Why do we let ourselves be victims of circumstances instead of creators of what we want? Why do we always look at what we *don't* have instead of what we *do* have? As a kid I remember getting 25 cents a week for an allowance—miserly even for those days! But the question I asked myself was not, "I can't buy anything I want with this quarter, so why bother?" Instead I asked the question, "What do I want and how can I get it?" The underlying assumption I had as a child was that I could choose how to spend my money.

In writing this book, I have noticed that whenever I declare I don't have time to write, I am correct. My schedule is jam-packed with appointments. And when I declare I do have time, I'm right about that too. I schedule my book-writing time as an appointment for myself. The underlying assumption is that I can choose what I do with my time.

Having "enough" time, money, resources, motivation, or anything else is totally a matter of cultivating the belief that you get to choose. What you do depends on what is most important to you. Staying healthy has nothing to do with limitations of money or time. Staying healthy requires you to prioritize your health. Those who prioritize health and fitness take the action required. Those who do not prioritize health and fitness do not take the action required. And both of these categories of people are choosing to say either yes or no to themselves.

Are you willing to say yes to yourself?

Diets Are Bad For You

*H*ave you noticed that most people who lose weight by dieting gain back their weight and usually regain more? Are you (or your weight-loss client) one of them? Dieting, especially yo-yo dieting, causes certain health risks and emotional/psychological risks in addition to the likelihood of not retaining your weight loss.

CBS News reports that 45 million Americans are on a diet, yet the Centers for Disease Control and Prevention reports that 68 percent of people over 20 years old are either obese or overweight. If we're all on diets, why are we still overweight? One reason is the phenomenon of rebound dieting, in which all of the weight loss, and sometimes more, is gained back once the diet is over. Nearly 65 percent of dieters return to their predieting weight within three years, according to Gary Foster, PhD, clinical director of the Weight and Eating Disorders Program at the University of Pennsylvania. Even worse are the statistics for dieters who lose weight rapidly, according to Wellsphere, a website sponsored by Stanford University. Only 5 percent of people who lose weight on a crash diet will keep the weight off.

Dropping pounds quickly doesn't mean you have dropped fat; it probably means you have lost water, which returns quickly once you resume normal eating.

In addition to the poor success rates, losing weight quickly carries serious health risks. Rapid weight loss that comes with crash dieting can make your bones frailer and denser, it can atrophy muscles, and it can wreak havoc with your immune system ... leaving you more susceptible to infections and illness. Your heart can also be damaged by extreme dieting. Cardiologist Isadore Rosenfeld, MD, warns that crash dieting can cause heart palpitations and even heart attacks. [1]

In addition to physical health risks, emotional/psychological risks of dieting include disempowering responses such as guilt, obsession, deprivation, binge and purge mentality, shame, secrecy, isolation, defiance, and so many more. Clients and family members have told me that the onset of their bulimia struggles occurred at a time when they were asked to cut certain foods out of their diet for health or weight reasons. The deprivation was too much to handle, so they ate the foods anyway and then vomited, beginning a destructive, addictive pattern, causing additional health complications.

Yo-yo dieting evokes similar, recurring indulgence/deprivation behavior patterns—like a manic-depressive merry-go-round experience which renders us euphoric when we are indulging and self-pitying when we are depriving ourselves. A diet mentality of either being on or off of it sets the stage for either believing "I'm good" or "I'm bad." People who binge and then feel guilty diminish their self-worth and self-confidence. Diet failures destroy confidence when the diet doesn't work or we can't stick with it. A poor self-image is exaggerated when we engage in yo-yo dieting, and it contributes to a mindset of poor self-worth. Living our lives with guilt or remorse about food contributes to a poor relationship with food, setting up a love-hate relationship with it that lasts a lifetime.

Diets are not the solution because food is not actually the problem. So how do we keep our weight off without the "D" word? I teach my weight-loss clients and my certified coaches to begin with our relationship to food. And then we look deeper to the real cause of overweight.

Exercise Doesn't Work

Most reputable weight-loss programs recommend exercise several times a week. Does this pattern resonate with you or your weight-loss client? We may have set our New Year's resolution to exercise every day for an hour. We may start out consistently, and then predictably we skip a day ... or two days. Before we know it, we are back to our pre-resolution exercise routine, whatever it may or may not have been. The reason exercise doesn't work in keeping our weight off is that we don't stick with it.

What is the problem here? Do we lack willpower, are we allergic to our own sweat, or did we decide fat is beautiful after all? None of the above! Overweight people can have interpretations of exercise as being hard, time-consuming, or boring. If we don't experience immediate results, we get discouraged. Exercise produces soreness, stiffness, and fatigue. Transitioning to an expanded exercise schedule requires intention, determination, and focus.

Question: Why would I want to do something long-term that is hard, boring, discouraging, painful, time-consuming, and messes up my regular routine?

Answer: I wouldn't! People do what brings pleasure and avoid what causes pain.

Good news! Our bodies are designed to move. Our bodies heal and flourish when we move. Our bodies mend and strengthen when we move. Our metabolism improves, our blood pressure normalizes, our menopause symptoms decrease, and our osteoporosis slows when we move. Our stress levels decline and our joy of life increases when we move. Our feel-good hormones of serotonin and dopamine rise when we move.

People who are immobile—like my former husband, who had a spinal cord injury, and our friend who had polio and is in a wheelchair—want to be mobile. They want to move. We all want to move, whether for physical reasons, to get around and go places, or for psychological and emotional reasons, to feel independent and free. We want to move when we're young, and we want to move even more as we age.

Since we really do want to move and since we really don't want pain, etc., how do we resolve this? I teach my weight-loss clients and my certified coaches to replace the word *exercise* with the word *movement* right from the start. Then I ask them to list their love, love, love movements as a homework assignment. Clients' lists include dancing, playing hopscotch, walking the dog, hula hooping, riding a bike in the park, making love, playing basketball and other games, doing yoga, hiking, and a variety of other enjoyable activities. When we remove pain and suffering from the context of exercise and then define movement as those activities we love to do, our ability to maintain the movement consistently is strengthened along with our bodies.

When I dropped 50 pounds in the 1990s, I did not exercise! I joined a ballroom dancing class and began preparing for amateur competitions and exhibitions. When our daughter Angela dropped her post-baby weight, she did not exercise. She began running with a friend, culminating in entering marathons around the country. Neither of us considered our routines "exercising," although technically we were doing so. But our context was about enjoyment, challenge, and participation in an activity we love.

What do you love, love, love to do that involves both movement and pleasure? What would it take to do more of it daily? What would you have to let go of in order to be consistent? What would you have to embrace? What would you have to believe?

Setting The Foundation

The curious paradox is that when I accept
myself just as I am, then I can change.
—Carl Rogers

If Discipline, Diets, and Exercise Don't Work, What Does Work?

The reason so many people are overweight these days goes much deeper than "I eat too much and don't get enough exercise." Those are just the symptoms. We use food for so many things besides a need for body fuel, which is indicated by physical hunger. I remember realizing *again* one Christmastime, as I baked a selection of homemade cookies, banana bread, and fudge to gift my loved ones, that I equated food with love. When Grandma Mary fixed lemon meringue pie, fried okra, fried pork chops, mashed potatoes, green beans, or chicken with dumplings for our visits as children, I knew she loved us. When my daddy gave us small boxes of chocolate candy for Valentine's Day or made his famous date nut roll, I knew he loved us. When my mother-in-law, Annalu, baked me those caramel pecan cinnamon rolls for my birthday and did so again when my father passed away many years later, I knew she loved me. Food equaled love in my mind! And this may be true for most overweight folks. Does food equal love to you?

Food can be a companion, a remedy for loneliness. Bryce, one of my weight-loss clients, confided to me that he noticed how sad he felt when he stuck to his food plan; his emotional experience was similar to that of losing a dear friend. The friend was the junk food he craved.

Physical hunger is our body's signal that we need fuel, but overweight people often confuse physical hunger with emotional hunger, which is not easily distinguished or recognized. Emotional hunger includes the need for socialization, the desire to be comforted, a camouflage to cover or suppress emotions, a distraction from boredom, a signal of fatigue, a remedy for stress, and a diversion from loneliness. When we think about or attempt removing the emotional foods that we love and instead only eat to fuel our bodies, inner turmoil ensues. We have built a relationship with food over the years. There will be consequences to pay, some uncomfortable, if we transform that relationship. We have habits to break. We must create new ways of viewing ourselves while embracing a new lifestyle. Relationships may change. In particular, we must begin to create a new relationship with ourselves, such as learning to love and accept ourselves and practicing exquisite self-care.

Ontology—the Missing Component

Weight loss and maintenance include more than food and exercise. These are only two of the three legs of the weight-loss tripod. The third leg, which is the missing component in most weight-loss programs, is called "Ontology." Maybe you have heard of this in other coaching programs or studies; most people are unfamiliar with the term, but herein lies the key to keeping your weight off forever.

Ontology is the science or study of being. It includes patterns, perspectives, and beliefs that we have created along our life journey, beginning in early childhood. We may be totally unaware of these. Ontology refers to the mental/emotional/psychological parts of human beings. So ontological coaching addresses the being, including these underlying perspectives, and is very powerful when combined with facilitative coaching—the doing. Facilitative coaching addresses the plan of action, accountability, the process you go through to get to your goal, what you "do." Ontological coaching addresses the mental/emotional/psychological aspects, how you "be."

My favorite illustration is the chocolate cake story. Let's say you've set your weight-loss goal as a New Year's resolution. You have your plan, and you have your two facilitative coaches: your nutritionist and your trainer at the gym. You even have a couple of friends to walk daily with you and to be accountability buddies with regard to your food.

But then something happens. And there you are at midnight eating the whole chocolate cake! Why are you doing this? The answers lie in the area of ontology. The Ontological Weight Loss Programs, along with this book, teach you what to do about it. Ontological coaching also provides positive, permanent shifts in how you relate to yourself, to your life, and to others.

So we begin your journey toward fabulous right now with some ontological training.

Addressing and transforming the underlying reasons for our food choices is a prerequisite to jumping off the weight-loss merry-go-round. If we don't get to the core reasons, eating will continue to be a war ... a struggle between deprivation and indulgence. Self-confidence will continue to dissolve into self-deprecation. Your body, which is designed to preserve your life, will become so confused that it won't know if you are in feast or famine mode and will retain fat, just in case. Without discovering and shifting your ontological sabotage patterns, you will find it harder to drop the weight and easier to put it back on as you age. It's a downward spiral.

Good news! What does work in weight loss and maintenance starts right here. You will learn the missing components and what to do to change permanently. The first step is to know who you really are—your authentic, core, essential self—as opposed to who you think you are or how you behave.

A Word on Willpower

How many times have we fallen off our program because of excuses or ignorance, without knowing why we did that? I remember declaring that I would be on a certain diet in the morning, and then by supper I had already eaten something off my plan. I also remember promising myself that I would get up early to exercise every day, but then before the week was over, I had broken my promise. In both of these circumstances, I wasn't even aware I had strayed off plan until afterward when I noticed my "reason" was really an excuse.

I have often criticized myself for being a lazy bum with no willpower. Have you ever said something like that to yourself? The truth is that I do have a lot of willpower in many areas, including food and exercise. When I began Latin dance competition and exhibition with a handsome, younger dance partner, I had no problem getting plenty of exercise and eating very healthy foods. When I wanted to fit into a smaller size for my wedding dress, I had no problem sticking to a low-carb regimen. When I found myself single after many years and on the "market" again, I easily worked out at the gym every night and cut back on my caloric intake. I suggest that you also have had experiences when your willpower was strong.

So where did the willpower go when those circumstances changed? Why didn't my weight or yours remain stable?

Willpower is not the answer! Willpower is defined as the "strength of will" or "strength of mind" and explains only a small part of why we do what we do or don't do. Your arm would tire if you tried to hold a heavy book in the air for an extended time without support, and your arm would finally drop the book, regardless of how much willpower you had. Just as your arm strength cannot last indefinitely, your willpower strength will also tire when you try to change a lifelong pattern without support. If you depend only on willpower, you will tire and drop off your program.

So let yourself off the hook! Thanks for being human! Willpower is not the answer. The answer lies in our predictable, automatic sabotaging behavior patterns, which must be changed at the core level and replaced with empowered behavior patterns. We must address real reasons and real solutions.

Why Do I Do What I Do?

When we are born, each of us brings to the world our own perfect little being. Our core essential being includes qualities that are intrinsic and love-based. We begin life with a pure, clean slate. Then in childhood, sometime before the age of seven, an event occurs that scares us, and we make it mean something. Maybe Mom didn't pay enough attention or Dad worked all the time, and we made it mean we weren't important. Or maybe Big Brother picked on us till we cried, and we made it mean that we were weak and wimpy.

The childhood meanings we made up translated into our deep fears. We didn't want to face those scary childhood fears. So in order to protect ourselves from them or to compensate for them, we created coping mechanisms and strategies, usually unconsciously, that were practiced and revised over the years until now, as adults, they have become automatic, predictable behavioral patterns.

As a child I made my parents' divorce and my mother's death mean that I was unlovable and not good enough. My small-child interpretation of their events was all about me. I didn't know this about me until years later. What I did know was that I binged on sweets a lot, but I never understood the connection between my bingeing and my meanings and interpretations about myself. This relationship was still at the unconscious level until years later. So even if you don't remember what happened in your young life or what interpretations you made about yourself at the time, be assured that this happened, even if it is still at the unconscious level.

These behavioral patterns dictate on an unconscious level how we deal with our perceived meanings from the circumstances we experience in life. Maybe the child who believed herself to be unimportant becomes a people pleaser. Maybe the child who believed himself to be weak and wimpy becomes a tough guy or rebel. Being unimportant, weak, and wimpy are the deep fears. People Pleaser and Rebel are protection strategies. We experience other emotions too, whether good, bad, or ugly. For example, the emotions of embarrassment, inadequacy, or self-criticism may emerge with the People Pleaser. The emotions of anger, resentment, or defiance might emerge with the Rebel.

Here is a recap showing how the process is created and continues to be reinforced:

- You are born as a pure little soul
- Something happens
- You make it mean something about you
- You experience a deep inner fear about yourself; for example, "I'm not good enough" or "I'm not lovable"
- You feel other emotions, along with your deep fear
- You develop protection strategy patterns to cope with the unwanted emotions
- Every time an unwanted emotion comes up, you practice, refine, and habitualize the strategy patterns you developed as a child
- You have created automatic and predictable (often unconscious) behavior patterns

If this normal cycle continues, you will run your life in predictable and automatic default mode, which I call protective default mechanism, and your weight will reflect it. If your behavior patterns are distinguished and transformed, you will create freedom for yourself and will drop your weight forever.

Your Protective Default Mechanism (PDM)

Although others have different names for it (such as Self-Defense, Survival Mechanism, and Pain Body), I call this model of experiencing fear, buffering by protective behaviors and strategies, and dealing with various emotions our Protective Default Mechanism or PDM. The behaviors that originated in childhood have now become automatic and predictable patterns. The default patterns reside within our comfort zone, not because they're really always comfortable, but because they're familiar, predictable, and automatic. We are "used to" behaving the way we do. We have created, adapted, and habitualized our reactions and behavior patterns over many years, so that the default patterns appear to occur in a normal, unconscious way. Many times, we have observed and adapted these default behavior patterns from our parents and other influential people while growing up. For instance, if my father was a perfectionist and workaholic to prove himself good enough, I might model him and adapt perfectionist or workaholic as my own Protective Default Mechanism patterns. Since these patterns are automatic, we may not be able to distinguish them or identify them as predictable patterns. We are too close to them to see them.

Most often we don't even recognize our deep fears, since we have worked so long at protecting ourselves from feeling those fears or because we never distinguished/identified them at all. We may not fully recognize our other emotions either. We may react to circumstances and automatically jump into our predictable behavior strategy patterns. If we are not aware of the protective defaults as behavior strategies, we might confuse them with who we *really* are—our authentic, core, essential self. But the Protective Default Mechanisms are not who we are; they are just what we do—patterns of strategies or behaviors— to protect ourselves from the deep (subconscious) fears.

We all have several Protective Default Mechanisms, which usually work together. For instance, if we distinguish that Mary's PDM patterns are "Anxious, People Pleaser, Anal, Perfectionist, and Workaholic," she will probably work long hours trying to impress her boss, get the project done right, and then worry about it after work hours. Once we become aware of a cycle and take a look at our own behavior patterns, it's pretty easy to identify them for ourselves. When I work with my clients, I can identify several patterns from their initial assessment and subsequent discussions. In addition, once they understand the process, with a little encouragement, they can identify their own protective patterns. When I coach couples, the spouse can usually add a few more to the list! What is one of your patterns that you know are automatic and predictable? Remember, this is not who you are; it's just what you do.

In working with my clients, I like to name the Protective Default Mechanism patterns in order to distinguish them as separate from the client. For instance, when we discover that Mary has developed People Pleaser as her pattern, we may name it "Penelope People Pleaser." If Bill has developed Rebel as his pattern, we may name it "Roger Rebel."

Another way I support clients in distinguishing their protective default mechanism patterns as behavior strategies is to use dramatic or crass words to make an impact. Instead of "Penelope People Pleaser," we might name Mary's pattern "Susie Suck Up" or "Barbie Brown Nose." Stronger words aid in our ability to remember the pattern and to notice when it shows up. Examples of patterns include the following: anal, overwhelmed, perfectionist, procrastinator, crazy, raging, airhead, anxious, scaredy-cat, control freak, loser, rebel, whiny baby, Nazi, ostrich, bag lady, stupid, and scattered.

One might recognize a Protective Default Mechanism pattern based on the internal self-talk or observation:

- Debby Denial or Pete Procrastinator says, "I won't think about this today."
- Nancy Nazi or Judgmental Judy says, "I am a loser!" or "I screwed up!"
- Ruby Rebel or Larry Outlaw says, "I'll show them!"
- Wendy Whiner or Quincy Quitter says, "I can't do this anymore!"

In weight loss, the PDM patterns emerge as saboteurs of our commitment. Mary's "Penelope People Pleaser" has difficulty saying no when a friend insists "…just eat the cookies this one time; I made them especially for you." Bill's "Roger Rebel" resists diet plans or exercise regimens which someone else has prescribed.

Our Protective Default Mechanism patterns are sly, cunning reactions. They operate subconsciously unless we are aware and conscious. Once we are aware and conscious of our default patterns, they remain until we choose and practice new ways of behaving. But our patterns don't easily change. Whenever we move from familiar to new ways of behaving, our Protective Default Mechanism says in effect, "Danger! This is outside my familiar comfort zone!" And our default strives to firmly remain the same and to keep us protected and safe.

A great example of how the Protective Default Mechanism affects our choices in weight loss came from my client Ann. Ann wanted to lose 50 pounds. Her automatic default pattern included Hilary Hopeless and Rene Resignation, which protected her from the fear that she was not good enough. When Ann made choices from these patterns of Resigned and Hopeless, she would quit. It appeared to be her decision, even though it was really an automatic default decision to quit. And all of this happened before anyone, including Ann herself, faced her fear that she was not good enough.

So Ann joined a popular weight-loss program and began the food plan, which excluded sugar. Before she arrived at the dinner party Saturday night, she decided not to have the dessert. But when the hostess served dessert, Hilary Hopeless and Rene Resignation talked Ann into eating it, because they implied, "Have the dessert, Ann. Why deprive yourself, when it won't make any difference? You never have and never will succeed at losing weight anyway."

Ann ate this dessert and then felt bad about herself and her lack of "willpower," so when she returned home, she ate a quart of ice cream to help her numb the emotions she did not want to feel—shame and guilt, based on her unconscious belief, "I have no willpower, so I must not be good enough." Ann's patterns of Hopeless and Resignation sabotaged her weight-loss commitment. This was familiar for Ann.

In contrast, after her transformative Ontological Weight Loss program, Ann believes that she is "good enough." She does not listen to or react to her automatic sabotaging voices of Hopeless and Resignation. Ann now makes different choices. She instead listens to the voices of her commitment and her weight-loss vision. Ann now makes empowered choices, such as:

- skipping dessert
- eating a bite of the dessert and then stopping
- eating and enjoying a serving of dessert without guilt, then returning to her plan
- adding additional exercise to burn off the dessert calories

The choices I make today will determine the rest of my life!
—Ginny Dye

How we do one thing is how we do anything. So whenever we are confronted with our Deep Fear, we automatically revert to familiar ways of coping. For instance, if Ann argues with her boss and is afraid of being fired, the fear of "not good enough" may emerge. And this fear, too scary to consciously consider, invokes the automatic and predictable pattern of eating sweets or drinking alcohol to suppress her fear. What about you? Do you eat or drink in the evening in response to a stressful day at work? Underneath may be your own fear of not being good enough.

The bigger your new possibility, which represents a huge change from the familiar comfort zone, the more your protective default mechanism dips into its arsenal to retrieve patterns and strategies to protect you from your deep perceived fears. This explains why so many public figures and spokespeople for weight-loss programs, as well as those of us in the general public, regain their former weight. They haven't done the inner, ontological work, so their predictable Protective Default Mechanism patterns eventually take control.

Remember, after years of fine-tuning, these are automatic and predictable behavior patterns, so you may not even be tuned in to your stimulus/response cycle. As you become more aware of your automatic and predictable strategies, you are able to then explore the deep fears underneath. Therein lies the power to shift our behaviors to ones that support our weight goals.

Authentic Self: If I'm Not My Authentic Self, Who Am I Really?

Regardless of how or when the Protective Default Mechanism exhibits itself, your core essential being remains solid and steady. PDM behaviors are like the surface of a lake during a storm, with whitecaps and turbulence, reacting to the elements. Your core essential self is like the serene bottom of the lake, calm and undisturbed by the weather above. Core essential self is called by many other names, including Essence, Core Being, Authentic Self, Essential Being, Higher Self, Presence, Consciousness, Spiritual Self, Wisdom, and Divine Self. We use the term "Essence" for our discussion purposes.

Essence is and always will be who you really are, the pure being of love you are—before you make circumstances mean anything about yourself. Your Essence is your authentic self. While we can readily see Essence in others, we often are not conscious of or able to identify our own Essence; yet understanding, identifying, and owning it provides a huge advantage in your weight-loss journey. When we make decisions from our authentic, essential self, we tend to choose wisely from the perspective of commitment, vision, and outcome. Then our Protective Default Mechanism sabotage patterns don't run the show. From Essence we facilitate our weight-loss success with velocity and passion

Practice Exercises/Assignments/Action

We have covered much information regarding the foundation of ontology! This information is a key component in understanding our ontological sabotage patterns and in understanding why we can't keep our weight off permanently. Remember, ontology is the most important leg of the tripod of successful weight maintenance: ontology, nutrition, and movement. We can diet and exercise until the cows come home, but unless we address the "who, why, and what" beneath the "how" of diet and exercise, we will not be able to maintain our weight.

Understanding is only part of the solution, however. To be successful in our weight-loss journey, we must take the next step: integrate this academic knowledge into our lives, so that in addition to understanding, we also practice and shift to the new default behavior patterns.

This is the process of transformation.

When I work with individuals and organizations, we go deeper into the process of integration and transformation. Therefore, all of our programs include exercises/assignments/action to further this process. In other words, we do the assignment, practice the new behaviors, and make permanent changes in our perception and behavior. I coach clients throughout the process. Because we are *practicing* new ways of being, seeing, and relating, we call these action steps/exercises/assignments "Practices."

By the way, if you resist, procrastinate, or talk yourself out of completing these Practices, note that the Protective Default Mechanism made the decision, not Essence. Often my clients make excuses that sound "reasonable" to them. Transformation brings up fears we didn't know we had, so remember that this is normal; your process is perfect. When my clients have any blocks in completing their assignments, I ask them, "What are you afraid of?" or "What's scary about doing them?" And we walk together through the obstacles.

Below are two practice areas that will enhance your awareness of who you are vs. what you do.

- Notice when you are in your Essence. This is who you are. In Essence you will show up in a positive, flowing way; for example, joy, empowerment, peace, love, confidence, security, wisdom, courage, etc.
- Notice when you are in a Protective Default Mechanism (PDM) pattern. This is NOT who you are; it is just what you do. In PDM, you will experience life in a disempowered way with perhaps resistance or struggle; for example, acting resentful, angry, obsessive, timid, insecure, scared, defensive, guilty, etc.

For additional practice action steps to integrate your academic learning into your reality, please refer to our *Lose Weight for Life Companion Workbook* or to our O.W.L. Weight Loss Programs.

Context Is Decisive

Webster's New World College Dictionary defines context as "the whole situation, background, or environment relevant to a particular event, personality, creation, etc." In other words, our context means our perception, perspective, or beliefs based upon our outlook. It's our relationship to the world. It's how we view ourselves and how we view circumstances and others.

The context, or perspective, we are using at any particular time is sometimes conscious and distinguished, but many times we are totally unaware of it. We often make decisions based on our context, even though we don't know we have done so. Imagine a fish in a tank, unaware of the water in which it swims. We are the fish; our context is the water.

Context can also be described as a filter, like wearing sunglasses. When we put on green sunglass lenses, we see the world through a green filter. At first we might recognize the greenness, but as time passes we forget that our world appears a little greener. Only when we remember we are wearing the green sunglasses or when we remove them do we realize the truth: The world is not as green as we thought.

Our beliefs are like these lenses, and they determine what we see, the decisions we make, and what actions we take. Cathy believed that she had inherited her weight problem from her family because they were all obese. This was her perspective, the way she saw her world, her context. Every attempt Cathy made to lose weight was doomed to fail from the outset because her actions were founded on the belief that nothing would work anyway. From the context of "this won't work," Cathy cheated on her food program and made excuses not to exercise.

Once Cathy distinguished through our coaching that her belief originated from a faulty underlying context, she realized that a more accurate explanation for her obese family included modeled and learned habits, such as overeating, inactivity, and stuffing down emotions. She saw that these habits could be changed. Cathy shifted her context about inheriting her tendency to gain weight and began to make decisions based on her commitment, not her former restrictive interpretation.

When our beliefs are not in alignment with our desires, we begin to manage our beliefs in hopes that something will change. Before she began coaching with me, Darlene believed that she needed to fix herself, that there was something wrong with her. Among other perceived faults, Darlene believed that she did not have enough willpower to successfully reach her goal weight. Consequently, she judged herself as bad and wrong. So she tried to manage those beliefs by starting one diet program after another, hoping something would change.

Darlene failed at every program she began. What she did not know was that the more she tried to manage her belief, the more "real" the belief became. After each failed diet, Darlene reinforced her beliefs that she could never succeed and it was all her fault. But the problem was not with Darlene. The problem was not with any particular diet. The problem was her belief.

The good news is that we can change our beliefs once we know what they are! We have the choice to believe what we want to believe. With coaching, Darlene gradually learned that there is nothing wrong with her. She learned to love and nurture herself. She realized that she could change her context with awareness and choice. Darlene replaced her yo-yo dieting with permanent weight loss.

Our beliefs, whether conscious or not, motivate us to take particular actions, and those actions lead to particular results. Cathy's belief that fat runs in her family led her to give up sooner every time she tried to release weight. Darlene's belief that she was flawed and had no will-power led her to try one program after another, hoping to fix herself. Both ladies had not recognized these underlying beliefs until, with our coaching, they began to look deeper for reasons (the real reasons) they could not drop the weight. They could then engage in the process of shifting context.

By the way, I shared Cathy's and Darlene's unconscious context; I had an overweight dad and grandmother and tried to fix myself. I fretted and worried because I believed I had inherited my family's obesity and could not change anything. I also believed that because my mother had killed herself, I must be unworthy and unlovable—I was flawed. So I went on every weight-loss program I knew of, including healthy and unhealthy ones. All the while, I strove to prove that my obesity wasn't inherited and that I wasn't doomed to failure. The more programs I tried and failed, the more my beliefs were validated and confirmed.

Attempting to lose weight with an undistinguished, disempowering context kept me on the merry-go-round of frustration and overweight. Within this world, I was always gathering evidence for that which I believed to be true. So when I thought obesity ran in my family, I saw all the evidence that convinced me it was true. When I thought that weight loss required willpower and that I didn't have enough willpower to succeed, I saw all the evidence to prove that true. And so it is with us all. We see through lenses of belief, and we then gather evidence that it must be true, thus validating and "proving" our belief ... until we change the belief.

Viewing ourselves with a disempowered context or belief makes it impossible to see anything else and, therefore, impossible to make empowered decisions and achieve results. What do your contexts make impossible for you ... permanent, easy weight loss and maintenance, perhaps? If you took off the glasses or filter of disempowering beliefs, what would be possible?

- As a practice exercise to identify and change context, notice a belief you have about your weight-loss progress that keeps you stuck. How could someone else interpret this differently in a more empowering way? Which of these two contexts will you choose to believe?

Nine Reasons You Can't Keep Your Weight Off

You have now learned three valuable foundational distinctions for your journey to successful, permanent weight loss:

1. Your sabotaging Protective Default Mechanism patterns, which explain why you fall off your program
2. Your Essence—your authentic self, which helps you to lose weight successfully through wise choices
3. Your context and beliefs, which explain how you see yourself in the world and why you succeed or do not succeed

Are you ready to learn the nine specific reasons that you cannot keep your weight off and what to do about them? Each of these reasons may be unconscious or conscious right now. Each one may be operating alone or it may be operating in conjunction with one or more of the other reasons. And each reason is based on the foundational information we have covered thus far.

Also, when any of these nine reasons show up for you with regard to your weight, they probably show up in other areas of your life as well, because how we do one thing is how we do everything. So when you have learned what to do about each one with regard to weight, you will also see benefits reflected elsewhere.

I'm excited to share these with you, as they mark the basis for my signature, proven methodology for teaching people how to achieve permanent weight loss.

Reason 1: Unmet Needs And Unexpressed Emotions

You are precious and good. Your process is perfect.
When you learn to love yourself with all your heart and
mind and body and spirit, you will experience the joy, peace,
and health that you desire. You are a perfect child of God.
God and I love you just the way you are!
—Janis Charlton Pullen

The Sabotage Pattern

When I was young, I learned, "Children should be seen and not heard" and "If you can't say anything nice, don't say anything at all." When my parents fought and divorced, I made it mean that anger caused people to leave me. When my stepmother was abusive to me and my sisters, I learned that my rage made it worse, so I became stoic. When I was a teenager, I heard and believed the song lyrics, "Big Girls Don't Cry." As a CPA in corporate America, I learned that emotions did not belong in the workplace. As a wife, I learned from my husband that the best way of relating with his mother was for me to "dial it down," meaning my "overexpressing" was uncomfortable for them both.

The common theme in these messages—and countless others we receive all the time—is that it is wrong and bad to express emotions. So to keep our emotions "in control" and heed these messages, we must do something to dissolve, stuff, transform, or replace them. My tactic was to stuff my emotions with food.

As the oldest child in a dysfunctional family, I played the role of the good girl. I noticed what was wrong and tried to fix it before it could cause problems. I worried about my younger sister, who always bore the brunt of the physical abuse. Basically, I learned to take care of other people's needs at the expense of meeting my own. In my relationships I always deferred to the other person's needs and wants. So you could say I stuffed my needs down the same way I stuffed my emotions down.

Stuffing as I did is common. Overweight people often don't recognize their own emotions or needs, they don't relate to them, or they have a context/judgment that they are selfish or wrong to try to fulfill their needs or express their emotions. However, the topic of needs and emotions is paramount to losing weight because we are not robots; we are human, and we do have needs and emotions! For your information, our emotions and needs are not going away! They are merely being stuffed down as we eat for comfort, for numbing out, for compensation for unmet needs, and for emotion management. Many times we also use other ways to stuff down feelings, such as alcohol, shopping, gambling, sex, and other compulsions. We stuff down our emotions and needs consciously and unconsciously as a predictable, automatic reaction … our PDM to the rescue!

Becoming expert at identifying emotions and needs is a powerful step to breaking out of this "Unmet Needs and Unexpressed Emotions" sabotage, the first key reason we can't keep the weight off. When we know what we feel, we can learn what else to do with those emotions besides eat. When we know what we need, we can learn ways to get our needs met. We no longer must automatically resort to eating or drinking as a way to hide from ourselves, and our weight begins to drop off automatically.

What Do I Need?

What do our human needs encompass besides air, water, and food? Consider the following:

- Empowerment Coach Anthony Robbins, in several of his books and CDs, identifies six fundamental and spiritual needs of human beings: Certainty, Significance, Love, Variety, Growth, and Contribution.[2]
- American psychologist Abraham Maslow proposed his theory of hierarchy of needs, which includes Physiological, Safety, Love/Belonging, Esteem, and Self-Actualization.[3]
- Twelve-step programs, such as Overeaters Anonymous and Compulsive Eaters Anonymous, define four areas where needs must be identified and resolved: Hungry, Angry, Lonely, and Tired (H.A.L.T.)[4]
- The O.W.L. Weight Loss Program: Your Once-in-a-Lifetime Solution, adds Boredom and Stress to the OA areas (H.A.L.T.B.S.). These are red flags signifying an undistinguished emotion or need.[5]

In our Ontological Weight Loss programs we discover various levels of needs, and we practice self-love by identifying and fulfilling our needs. We also recognize emotions and honor those as a part of our authentic, human experience. We start with basics and then expand to deeper areas. We explore physical, mental, emotional, and spiritual areas of needs. We also look at areas regarding relationships and lifestyle, which include family, career, and finances.

Edie was someone people could always count on. She was there for everyone when they needed her help or her time. The problem was that Edie didn't even know that her own needs were not being met, because she didn't think about what she needed. So instead of asking for a hug or asking for help, she powered through by herself. When I asked Edie to reflect upon what she needed several times during the day by asking herself, "What do I need right now?" as a practice, she responded as if I had spoken to her in Greek. She tried it anyway and realized she was stuffing down her needs with cookies and coffee drinks. Once Edie identified her needs, she could focus on getting them met instead of stuffing them.

Fran was very busy taking care of a husband and two children. When she first began her coaching program with me, she was tired, angry, and resentful; she complained that she had given up her "life" to be a homemaker. Once Fran realized that she was worth fulfilling her own needs first, she resumed going to yoga classes, allowing herself alone time, and asking for help from her husband and others. She became energized and happy again, loving to spend time with her family. As a bonus, she began dropping her excess weight!

Do you know what you need? Where do you deny or subordinate your needs? How does this affect you? How does this affect those around you?

What Do I Feel?

In addition to needs, emotions are tricky for overweight people. You may not be surprised at how many people don't know how to describe what they are feeling. On a coaching call a client might say, "I'm emotional," and when I ask what the emotion is, they are not sure. Even if a client can identify the specific emotion, then she or he wants help to fix it. Emotions are frightening for people. We learn early in life that it's not OK to cry or to yell. We stuff our grief for so long that we are afraid to cry; it might open the floodgates and never stop. We stuff our anger for so long that we are afraid to release it; if we did, we might kill someone. Some of my weight-loss clients have not felt emotion for years. They ate to suppress the feelings.

It isn't only the "negative" emotions we want to avoid, such as anger, resentment, jealousy, or hatred. We also fear the "positive" ones, such as too much joy, compassion, or love. We make up stories that those good feelings may not last, or are not real, or have a price to pay. For example, do you know anyone who was afraid to fall in love for fear of being hurt?

In the O.W.L. Weight Loss Programs our required reading list includes *The Gift of Our Compulsions* by Mary O'Malley.[6] This book gives a brilliant explanation of the process we have taken to box our scary emotions and store them in the basement of our metaphorical home. Since our scary emotions must be felt sooner or later, they come up the stairs to find us. Frightened by them, we attempt to escape by ascending to the attic. Eventually we eat to avoid the emotions, or we engage in another compulsion to keep them away (shopping, alcohol, drama, etc.).

The good news is that, as mentioned earlier, we are human beings, not robots. We all have emotions, whether we want to face them or not. The emotions are not the problem. Rather how we view them (context) and how we process them become the challenge to resolve.

I like to use the metaphor of clouds when coaching clients on expressing their emotions. Clouds can be ominous, dark thunderstorm clouds, black and scary. They can be cute, white, puffy clouds that look like little lambs. They can last a long time, as they did with Tropical Storm Gilda in the 1970s, which brought three weeks of solid rain with no break and filled our car with water. Or they can be gone in a few moments as the wind scatters them and blows them away.

If we view our emotions as clouds (context), we know they are here for a while and then gone. There is nothing to "do" about them. We only notice them and "be with" them. As the alien Borg said (in the television program "Star Trek: The Next Generation") to Captain Jean-Luc Picard, "Resistance is futile!"[7] Likewise, resistance is futile for us regarding emotions. The more we resist or deny our emotions, the more they chase after us and the more we perceive that we must eat or otherwise indulge in compulsions to resist and numb out. On the other hand, when we stop resisting and "be with" our emotions, honoring and allowing them to be OK, guess what? They evaporate. They no longer control either us or our eating patterns.

When we resist the practice of noticing and expressing our emotions or when we resist the practice of identifying and fulfilling our own needs, we slowly kill ourselves, both physically and emotionally.

Consider the metaphor of the oxygen mask. At the beginning of each flight, the attendant instructs passengers to put the oxygen mask on themselves first and then to assist other passengers, including children. Why? If you don't get the oxygen to yourself first, you cannot help anyone else; you will be dead!

Translated to life, if you are not taking care of yourself first, how can you help others? Taking care of yourself includes fulfilling your needs and expressing your emotions. Furthermore, if you are not taking care of yourself, you cannot build a solid foundation for creating anything—your health, your career, your relationships, your finances, or your future.

Fred was taught by his father that boys who cry are sissies and that anger becomes dangerous when out of control. Fred's father never cried, and he hurt people, including Fred, when angry. Fred learned early to shut down all his emotions to be on the safe side. Instead of expressing feelings, Fred ate. He never learned that emotions are part of being human. He never learned that "feeling" is not the same as "acting," meaning we can feel anger without doing anything about it; for example, hitting or yelling. Once Fred learned that he could identify, accept, and "be with" his emotions, he experienced compassion for himself and reduced his numbing-out habit with food. Fred dropped 40 pounds with this insight alone.

Scary emotions like anger or loneliness are not the only ones we resist and stuff down with food. At the opposite end of the feeling spectrum, delightful emotions like joy or passion are numbed or suppressed when beyond our comfort zones. Numbing the "bad" also numbs the "good" emotions.

I knew Gabby was out of touch with her emotions even before she hired me. In our first strategy session together, when I asked her to visualize herself at her ideal weight and to tell me how it would feel, she had no clue how to feel anything, much less verbalize it. She had closed off her ability to feel excitement in many areas, not just weight. Gabby had conditioned herself to be protected from hope followed by disappointment, from love followed by heartache, and from joy followed by suffering. Food, wine, and shopping protected Gabby by substituting "highs" for her suppressed emotions—all of them!

Many times my clients confuse emotional hunger, which has been suppressed and not identified, with physical hunger. When we do not distinguish emotional from physical hunger, we eat for the wrong reasons. We eat to fill the emotional void instead of or in addition to eating to fill the physical hunger.

In what ways do you confuse or collapse emotional hunger and physical hunger in one clump, rather than distinguishing them as separate? In what ways could you deal with emotional hunger rather than with food, alcohol, or other compulsions?

What to Do About It

The way to resolve the first reason you can't keep the weight off is Presence and Awareness. Have you noticed that the practice assignments I suggested earlier include the action step of *noticing*? No accident here! In order to shift out of the sabotage of Unmet Needs and Unexpressed Emotions, what we need to do to drop our weight and keep it off forever is a shift to "Presence and Awareness."

Presence involves "being here now." We give up numbing out, being distracted, dishonoring our intuition, and being on autopilot. We give up our PDM's message to live in the past with regret or guilt. We give up our PDM's message to live in the future with anxiety and apprehension. Living in a past or future context gives the PDM something to do: to protect you with its strategies. It has no job if we focus on being present. With Presence we give attention to what we are doing, how we feel, what we need and want, who we are being, and how we are relating to the world ... right now. We become more intentional and less mechanical. We don't live in a context of past regret or future anxiety. We are present (aware) in the present (moment).

The clock is running. Make the most of today.
Time waits for no man.
Yesterday is history. Tomorrow is a mystery. Today is a gift.
That's why it is called the present.
—Origin Uncertain

Awareness implies that we are alert, mindful, and cognizant. It implies that we notice attentively and purposefully. When we become conscious observers of ourselves and of our behavior, we notice, honor, and "be with" our emotions. We notice, distinguish, and fulfill our needs. Sometimes we don't like what we experience, see, or feel; nevertheless, awareness provides the pathway to change. If we are oblivious or in denial, we are just like an ostrich with its head in the ground and have no power or means for growth and transformation.

Tammy, one of my weight-loss clients, reported in her first month of the program, "I sure am doing a lot of noticing these days! I see things I never saw before." Even before she started her food plan, Tammy began noticing how she felt when she ate, why she ate when she did, and how different foods affected her body and mood. Tammy realized that she craved certain foods during emotional times and during periods of boredom. Simply by practicing "Presence and Awareness," Tammy was able to identify what she really needed and felt. Through our coaching together, she was also able to go even deeper and to ask for what she needed.

Susan reported that because of her noticing practices in the early weeks of her O.W.L. program, she dropped eight pounds even before beginning her Level 1 Food Plan.

Ted had been worried that he would, in his words, "screw up again" and gain his weight back. He had been figuratively throwing up (vomiting) his past onto his future. When he realized in our coaching sessions that this old context created a domino effect in terms of discouragement and resignation, he created a new context for possibility and success. Ted began focusing on and sticking to his program one day at a time.

Many of my O.W.L. weight-loss clients consistently release five or more pounds right off the bat, as Susan did, without changing anything else in their lives except being present and aware—simply noticing. They notice WHAT they are eating, they notice WHY they are eating (Hungry, Sad, Angry, Lonely, Tired, Bored, Stressed, etc.), and they notice WHEN they are eating. In the process, they then begin to release the weight. Awareness is powerful.

I often ask my clients to practice the "Conscious Eating" exercise I learned at a seminar, "Journey to the Boundless," conducted by physician, speaker, and author Deepak Chopra in Irving, Texas, in 1995. Here are my notes on conscious eating from that seminar:

1. Eat in silence
2. Look at your food
3. Thank the providers of your food (God, nature, preparers, etc.)
4. Have an intention to notice your intention to …
   a. Pick up the food
   b. Notice the texture and taste
   c. Chew
   d. Swallow
   e. Feel the sensation in your stomach

You will become aware of the physiological changes in your body. Your body will tell you which foods are best for you.

Take hot water with lemon every half hour to detoxify or lose weight.

This practice of Conscious Eating makes eating more pleasurable and fulfilling, rather than mindless and compulsive. Dr. Chopra has written a book with the same name as the workshop I attended, *JOURNEY TO THE BOUNDLESS: Exploring the Intimate Connection Between Your Mind, Body and Spirit.*[8]

To enhance your mindful eating practice, I also suggest you ask these two questions before putting anything into your mouth:

"What am I feeling right now?"

"What do I need right now?"

Usually, the answer is not about food at all, unless it's from physical hunger. It so, then healthy food will satisfy. Hunger from feelings and needs is not satisfied with healthy food. Emotional hunger drives us to unhealthy eating. When feelings and needs are identified and addressed in a manner appropriate to the real cause, we don't have to use food to fill them. And the weight drops off.

No one can listen to your body for you.
To grow and heal, you have
to take responsibility for listening to it yourself.
—Jon Kabat-Zinn

Reason 2: Sacrifice/Entitlement

You yourself, as much as anybody in the entire universe, deserve your love and affection.
—The Buddha

The Sabotage Pattern

*H*ave you ever been on a diet, being really disciplined, and then Friday night at dinner you declare that you *will* have the wine, the fried potatoes, the rolls, and/or the dessert because you have been so good all week? Or have you ever tolerated a friend or relative who was driving you crazy, and then when they left, or even beforehand, decided to reward yourself with food? Just recently I took myself through a liver/gall bladder cleanse which involved giving up certain foods and then fasting for 24 hours. Afterward I wanted to eat everything in sight!

These instances, including the story of my mother-in-law's homemade caramel pecan cinnamon rolls, represent the second reason we can't keep our weight off: the sabotage pattern that I call "Sacrifice and Entitlement." I also call this pattern "Deprivation and Indulgence." Those who are giving excessively of themselves or are not getting their own needs fulfilled might be prone to the Sacrifice/Entitlement sabotage. Those who are stifling their emotions instead of expressing them might also be prone to this sabotage pattern.

When we held our original strategy session, Helen told me she could not stick to a diet because food was the only area in which she could indulge herself. She sacrificed in so many other areas of her life that she could not and would not give up eating whatever she wanted. She predicted that giving up those foods would be too much sacrifice for her, and she felt entitled to the pleasure of eating. She had not yet learned how to get out of the Sacrifice/Entitlement pattern, proven by her extra 76 pounds.

Whenever I participated in restrictive or crash diets, skipped meals, binged and then starved, or otherwise experienced anorexic tendencies, I evoked an undistinguished Sacrifice/Entitlement sabotage pattern. During a period in my life I ate very little and lost way too much weight, so much, in fact, that co-workers were concerned about me and brought it to my attention. I was in the sacrifice mode during the week, barely eating anything. Then on weekends I shifted to the entitlement mode, during which I ate Häagen-Dazs butter pecan ice cream.

Ultimately and predictably, I later regained the weight and became obese. Yet, I retained the belief that if I starved myself all day, I could have whatever I wanted in the evening. Even recently, while I maintain a healthy weight, whenever I have tried liquid meal replacements or cleansing fasts, my starve/binge tendencies emerge and I think I "deserve" to overeat afterward. This is another example of the Sacrifice/Entitlement pattern. (Bulimia sufferers often run this pattern with the addition of vomiting the food afterward.)

Where are you sacrificing in your life—with food, emotional fulfillment, settling for less, putting up with someone or something, or any other area? How does that sacrifice impact you? How does it impact your weight loss or weight maintenance?

What to Do About It: Two Pillars of Success

When I work with organizational or individual clients, we address the climate and culture in which they are immersed. We look at exquisite well-being and integrity as key components in maintaining healthy weight. My clients have learned that they cannot accomplish anything with excellence if their foundational practices (pillars of success) of well-being and integrity are weak. It's like trying to build a skyscraper on quicksand instead of rebar and concrete.

If your well-being and integrity are below 80%, you will have less than 80% effectiveness in accomplishing results. It would be like making a grade in school of C or below, with no chance of making the dean's list. Boosting your well-being and integrity to the 90%–100% range empowers you to shift the Sacrifice/Entitlement sabotage once and for all. Maintaining well-being and integrity standards equates to having strong foundational pillars of success upon which to build your results.

Well-Being—What Difference Does It Make?

Well-being, or self-care, correlates with resilience, the ability to recover quickly from life's "road bumps." Whenever a client reports a block or diversion from their weight plan, I know a well-being decline exists. Needs and feelings have not been fulfilled or honored. This is a common problem with overweight people.

One reason we don't honor our needs and feelings is that we have learned somewhere in the past that it would be selfish to do so. We may have been taught that it's more blessed to give than to receive. Maybe we have given our energies and nurturing to a spouse and/or children, without leaving time for ourselves. Maybe we have been taught, as I was, that we were selfish when we took care of ourselves or that others take precedence.

We have essentially collapsed the meanings of Selfish and Self-Care into one word, "Selfish." Did you know that in many non-English languages there are two distinct words to describe "Selfish"? One word means greedy and mean. The other means taking care of one's self. Our language is not so clear. That's a problem, because we assume the self-care interpretation is bad. And it's not! It's crucial to being your highest and best, which includes dropping excess weight.

Well-being, or self-care, is determined on a personal basis in four main areas: physical, mental, emotional, spiritual, plus any other areas you deem to be supportive. Taking care of yourself ensures energy, vitality, power, and good mood. It recharges your batteries. It revives your lifeblood. As aforementioned, well-being also improves resilience. Flight attendants instruct us to put the oxygen mask on ourselves first in case of emergency and then on others, including children. If we don't follow those instructions and the oxygen level drops, we would die before we could assist others. So put the oxygen mask on yourself first in your life by seeing that you give yourself exquisite care.

Ingrid was a model client during her O.W.L. Weight Loss Program, Levels 1–3. She dropped 50 pounds within six months and has kept it off since. However, in fine-tuning and maintaining her Level 4 O.W.L. Lifetime Plan, she often went on binges of "exception" food, the food items she considered treats rather than healthy.

When we delved more deeply into her triggers, the causes for her to binge, we found that each time she did so, her well-being was very low. When she increased her attention to well-being, her ability and her desire to adhere to her Lifetime Plan increased accordingly.

Those who think they have not time for bodily exercise will sooner or later have to find time for illness.
—Edward Stanley

What are the elements to consider to elevate your well-being? Physically, you might look at elements such as nutrition, water, sleep, exercise, relaxation, or massage. Mentally, you might consider brain stimulation like reading, crossword puzzles, stimulating conversation or debate, or learning a new language. Emotionally, you could explore avenues of emotional expression, family and social connection, praise and appreciation, or laughter. Spiritually, you might include quiet time, meditation, prayer, reflection, or being in nature. Many well-being activities fall into more than one category. For instance, music could be both emotional and spiritual, and quiet time could be physical, emotional, and spiritual. Attending to financial matters could be both emotional and mental.

What are five things that would improve your well-being on a daily basis? Would you be willing to include them each day as a priority?

Integrity—More than Being Honest

Integrity is the second foundational pillar of success, along with Well-Being, required to shift the Sacrifice/Entitlement sabotage pattern and accomplish permanent weight-loss results. Integrity can be defined as honesty, truth, honor, and reliability. In the world of coaching, Integrity is synonymous with a state of being "whole and complete, no parts broken." Consider a circle made with your two forefingers touching and your two thumbs touching. This circle is in integrity. But if you disconnect your two thumbs, the circle is out of integrity.

Integrity includes a broader version of our honesty in ways we may not yet have identified. I want to emphasize that for our purposes, integrity means "whole and complete, no parts broken." It means being in alignment with our authentic self—our Essence. When I was working in a college cafeteria, bussing tables, washing dishes, and plucking feathers off holiday turkeys for a minimum wage, I was out of integrity with my true life and business purposes. When I have an argument with my husband, I am out of integrity until I become "complete" by talking it out (and in my case, usually apologizing to him). When I harbored rage and blame toward my stepmother, I was out of integrity with my Essence of love and compassion.

When we harbor resentments or judgments, have nagging unfinished business, work or live in a messy environment, break promises to ourselves, behave from our PDM patterns, or keep secrets, we are out of integrity with our authentic, powerful self. If we have repressed emotions, unmet needs, or an unfulfilled purpose, we are also out of integrity with ourselves. Being in integrity with ourselves empowers and strengthens us. Being out of integrity with ourselves drains us of energy consciously or unconsciously. So we have to compensate; overweight people compensate with food.

Jenny realized that keeping secrets from her husband about how much money she spent on clothes was eating her up, meaning she felt guilty and ashamed. To cope with those feelings, Jenny turned to salty and sweet snacks on her way home from shopping to numb out, and she hid her purchases from hubby, which exacerbated the guilt. Once she discovered through our coaching the impact of secrets on her integrity, and consequently her weight, Jenny was able to clean up the deceit and get back into personal integrity.

The best way to maintain integrity, being whole and complete, is to notice where you are incomplete and take action to correct it. This is not a time to take out a big stick with which to beat yourself. This is a time to analyze, "What is so?" "What is missing?" "What is next?" Use a little compassion, or a lot of compassion.

Here are some areas to consider as you choose how to strengthen your integrity as a pillar of weight-loss success:

- Keeping promises to yourself and others
- Returning phone calls
- Maintaining neat personal and work environments
- Sticking to your plan—food, movement, well-being checklist, etc.
- Cleaning up relationships through conversation, compassion and forgiveness
- Finishing tasks

- Following your schedule
- Communicating openly and directly
- Expressing your emotions
- Being intentional—actions and thoughts in alignment with your commitment
- Tracking "what's so" on your weight and food tracking sheets

> *Be impeccable with your word.*
> *Don't take anything personally.*
> *Don't make assumptions.*
> *Always do your best.*
> —Don Miguel Ruiz[9]

- What is one area in which you are out of integrity (not whole and complete)? What is one step you can take today to regain your integrity in this area?

> *We are what we repeatedly do. Excellence, then,*
> *is not an act, but a habit.*
> —Aristotle

Reason 3:
Protection And Fear
Of Intimacy

There is a presence within you that has never suffered.
It has not been touched by anything you have experienced.
It has never achieved anything or cared to.
It is joyful for no reason. It has no problems.
It has been with you your entire life.
It is with you right now.
It is who you most deeply are.
—Jan Frazier, Zen Teacher

The Sabotage Pattern

*I*n reason #1 we discussed the Protective Default Mechanism as a set of behavior patterns or strategies that we created early in life to protect us from perceived fears of not being good enough, lovable, etc. The need for the PDM implies that we have something to hide and that we desire protection. The third reason we can't keep our weight off embodies the unconscious response to intimacy, meaning close familiarity and understanding. The mindset behind this sabotage pattern is, "If you find out the truth about me, you will not respect or love me anymore, and you will leave." How does this affect our weight?

Many people, especially overweight people, believe that they are flawed and must live up to an image, put on a front, or wear a mask in order to be accepted, respected, or valued. These folks are afraid that if others knew the truth about them (intimacy), they would surely be criticized and ultimately lose love or respect. They either recoil from conflict or they engage in conflict as a distancing strategy. When people try to hide their authentic selves from others for fear of being hurt, they often do so by being inauthentic, passive-aggressive, or uncommunicative rather than being authentic, assertive, direct, transparent, and open. They either shrink from difficult relationships or conversations, or they present a façade, instead of letting others see who they are and what they think. Some may become aggressive or confrontational, pushing others away in order to avoid closeness and honesty in relationships. Another protective strategy people utilize is failure to set or uphold clear-cut boundaries, as they try to fit in or please others. When any of these strategies emerge, the result equates with being a fraud. Fraud is not in alignment with who we are, so we have to do something to compensate. Compulsive eating, drinking, shopping, and so on, are predictable compensating behaviors.

When Grace hired me to help her lose 45 pounds, I noticed that she accommodated others in every way, including me in scheduling our coaching appointments. Grace was deathly afraid of criticism and of people not liking her. She was sweet and polite. She never disagreed with anyone, even if she had different opinions. Grace swallowed her anger, frustrations, and disappointments, not wanting to create waves or appear negative. She did everything that others asked her to do, so that no one would criticize her. Grace's worst nightmare was confronting conversations, so she stuffed all negative feelings and reactions by eating in order to feel better.

Howard, an executive with a Fortune 500 company, hired me to help him improve his relationships with his direct reports. He had noticed a lack of openness and trust, both with him and also between members of the group. During our coaching he discovered that his insecurities about being a "good enough" leader caused him to behave aggressively, with a "king of the mountain" mentality. He thought if he showed strength and judgment, people would respect him and his leadership. In adopting this behavior, Howard tried to prove his worth to his people, but he was really trying to prove his worth to himself.

The strategy of gruffness made Howard appear unapproachable, even though his authentic nature was kind and loving. So he unknowingly set an example for his people to be gruff, judgmental, and guarded. Oh, and I should mention that Howard was 50 pounds overweight as a result of trying to fill the gap between who he really was and the role he was playing ... stuffing the feelings of fraud.

When we fear intimacy, we create separation by withholding our true nature. To fill the gap, we overeat, and it's usually done unconsciously. Grace's mask of positivity created separation because people didn't really know who she was—her thoughts and emotions. Howard's mask of grouch separated him from his people and taught them to do the same. Both Grace and Howard were not showing up authentically for fear of disrespect or loss of love, so they ate to compensate.

We usually don't even know how or when our Protection and Fear of Intimacy sabotage is happening. There are several ways to notice it. When I work with executives and entrepreneurs, they learn to distinguish and understand the causes of the sabotage pattern and how to change.

- Notice where you tend to cover up, hide out, or push others away. Do you keep excess weight as a part of this protection strategy? What is scary about intimacy?

A few years ago I decided to have a total makeover—clothing, makeup, hair, and jewelry ... the whole shebang. When my consultant asked questions about my preferred style, I realized that for each stage of my career evolution I had assumed a different persona. The real me was masked. I had no preferred style because I was always playing a role.

For instance, as a CPA I wore navy, gray, and black tailored suits with pearls. But as a Mary Kay Senior Sales Director I wore excess everything, including bright colors, glitzy jewelry, big hair, and wild accessories. As a ballroom and Latin dancer, I wore a lot of black outfits, rhinestone-studded costumes, false eyelashes, and excessive makeup. Some might say I was "dressing for success" for each of these roles. As a life and business coach, I wasn't sure what to wear. There was no mold into which to fit myself. The truth was that I had taken on other people's perceptions of what was correct dressing because I was too insecure in my own identity. So the clothes and makeup became the mask behind which I hid. Since "how we do one thing is how we do anything," this Protection and Fear of Intimacy sabotage pattern showed up in other areas too. For instance, I never shared my opinions regarding politics or religion. I frankly did not allow myself to have opinions.

The sabotage pattern of Protection and Fear of Intimacy was exemplified in several episodes of the television program "What Not to Wear" when Stacy and Clinton's makeover clients dressed in clothing that hid their true selves. Clown attire, hooker-looking clothes, little girl T-shirts, and clothing printed with cow emblems are examples of ways to hide out, because other people see the covering and not the true nature or persona.

What to Do About It—Three Areas

In order to dissolve reason #3—the sabotage pattern of Protection and Fear of Intimacy—there are three areas to address: trust, communication, and managing the reactive PDM.

Trust—Self, Others, Spirit, and Circumstances

The first area is Trust. We fear intimacy—that is, letting people get too close to us—because we don't trust with regard to our relationships with ourselves, others, spirit (the Divine, God, Higher Power, the universe), or circumstances.

Trusting ourselves means knowing we will stand up for ourselves, that we will keep our promises to ourselves, and that we will notice and honor our intuition and wisdom. We can count on ourselves to take care of us. We trust ourselves to set and maintain appropriate boundaries with others. We respect and honor ourselves. Trusting myself was not always easy. For instance, I once ignored an intuitive thought to call a friend, and later learned that she had been in need of emotional support. I have rationalized that a marketing idea was wrong and later learned that it was perfect. I have since learned to trust myself—to listen and act upon the messages from my gut and my heart.

Trusting others means that we give the gift of trust whether others have earned it or not. I'm not referring to a stranger in a dark alley here. I'm referring to the people in your day-to-day life. Trusting others means we assume the best about people and give them the benefit of the doubt, instead of being cynical, suspicious, critical, and distrustful. We trust that others can handle whatever we have to say to them, so we are not afraid to be honest. We trust that others will take care of themselves, as we take care of ourselves. I had difficulty trusting others. I clearly remember the mantra my dad often recited, "If you want something done right, do it yourself." I had also created a childhood belief that I could not count on anyone, since my mother left me, my dad worked all the time, and my stepmother was the wicked witch of the west. Whew! With those lessons in place, no wonder I had trouble trusting others.

Trusting spirit, which is our Divine connection, implies that we believe we are in a loving, nurturing world, held with compassion, and seen as our highest and best selves. We know that everything is for our highest good. We invite and receive inspiration from a source larger than ourselves. We sense the connection of all. We follow Divine Guidance rather than dismissing the idea of it. When we are angry at spirit/God, we work it out, instead of abandoning or ignoring that relationship. This was also a difficult area for me. I was furious with God for my parental situation. Why didn't God watch out for me and nurture me? Why didn't God give me a happy childhood? Why did God disappear when I needed help?

Trusting circumstances means that we believe that "the process is perfect." It means that we see the good in everything that happens to us, even if it's just to become more compassionate or to learn something. Trusting circumstances requires that we remain in the present context, being here now. It requires that we view the past as experiential learning and as a contribution to our growth. And it requires that we view the future as positive and possibility. Obviously, my ability to trust the circumstances was diminished, since I couldn't easily trust others or God. In order to trust circumstances, I had to give up resentments stemming from my past. I had to look for the blessings. I had to learn to forgive. What would you have to give up for this "process is perfect" belief to exist? What would you have to take on?

My life is but a weaving
Between the Lord and me.
I cannot choose the colors
He weaveth steadily.

Oft times He weaveth sorrow;
And I, in foolish pride,
Forget He sees the upper,
And I the underside.

—Author unknown

Trusting ourselves, others, spirit, and circumstances are all related, because the choice is yours—the choice to give the gift of trust. Without that gift, the Protection and Fear of Intimacy sabotage pattern prevails. We behave from a context of fear and suspicion. We eat to fill the gap, soothe the soul, or numb the mind. We are out of integrity and alignment with our true authentic selves. And we usually don't even know what is happening underneath.

Grace, afraid of confronting conversations, had been frustrated with her roommate's messy habits and was afraid that if she voiced her frustration, he would become angry and move out. But she needed the income. She worried and fretted about this, often turning to wine in the evenings to numb her disgust at the mess. When she practiced giving the gift of trust to her roommate, believing that he could be understanding and compassionate, Grace discovered that they could have a congenial conversation and work things out. She also cut back on drinking for "medicinal purposes."

Humans are designed to crave relationship and intimacy. Ask any of my single clients who want to be married, or ask any of my clients who are in unfulfilling relationships! Lack of trust exacerbates sabotage pattern #3—Protection and Fear of Intimacy. When we are separate and distant from ourselves, others, spirit, and/or circumstances, we eat to fill the void or we numb out in other ways.

- What is one way you can give the gift of trust to yourself, to another person, or to your Divine Connection? What positive difference might that make for you?

Communication: Including Setting Boundaries and Being Heard

The second area to address in resolving Sabotage #3 is Communication, including Setting Boundaries and Being Heard. You may have reflected on how trusting yourself, others, spirit, and circumstances would change your communication, as it did for Grace. If you gave the gift of trust in any of these areas, what would you say that you don't say now? If you trusted yourself to be bold and trusted the other person to hear you, would you ask for what you want more readily and without hesitancy? If you trusted yourself to know what you need and trusted the other person to handle whatever came up, would you have the courage to set firm boundaries for yourself and to keep them? Would you voice your opinions or disagreements more readily? Would you stop settling, caving in, and avoiding? How could empowered communication enhance your relationships? How would it affect your relationship to food?

I teach my clients how to make and respond to requests, rather than making demands or complaining. Requests can be accepted, declined, or counter-offered. Adding a "please" to the sentence does not make it a request. A request includes a voice intonation of curiosity and an actual question, not a demand or blunt statement.

> *A complaint is an unexpressed request.*
> —Janis Pullen

I can request of my daughter, "Would you be willing to take out the garbage right after dinner?" or I can demand, "Take out the garbage!" The request empowers us both and increases the likelihood that she will comply without resentment. A request gives her the choice to respond with a yes, a no, or a counter-offer, such as, "I will, but may I do it tomorrow morning instead?"

I can request of my husband, "Would you be willing to help me with this?" or I can complain, "Why do I always have to do everything myself?" The request empowers us both and increases the probability that I will receive the help instead of a complaint that falls on deaf ears.

I enjoy teaching my clients the difference between communicating from their Essence versus from their PDM. They find when communicating from Essence that they relate to others with compassion instead of judgment. They also find that empowered, Essence-based communication is more likely to result in being heard. Empowered communication begins with a mindset of being "at cause" or proactive. Consider the proactive intentions of these words as a basis for communication: dedication, intention, possibility, proposal, promise, and decision.

In contrast, speaking with a mindset of being "at effect" is a reactive, victim context. It does not result in powerful or effective communication. When we speak from a victim context, people tune out or become defensive. The very things you want communicated become buried or blurred. Consider the victim/reactive intentions of these words as a basis for communication: cynicism, excuses, manipulation, judgment, and blame.

Another vital element in communication is the ability to set and keep boundaries for yourself. Are you a self-described pushover or wimp? Do other people infringe on your time, money, or emotions? Do others talk you out of your own opinions? Do you have trouble sticking up for yourself? If you answered affirmatively to any of these questions, the chances are good that you don't set and keep strong boundaries for yourself. Begin now by first determining your standards and preferences regarding what works and what doesn't work for you. In other words, determine what you want and what you don't want. Then let people know what those are, and stick to them.

Maintaining your boundaries strengthens your courage, self-worth, self-respect, and confidence. Boundaries, along with trusting yourself, others, and spirit, allow us to communicate at a deeper level with authenticity, clarity, and transparency. Consequently, we don't automatically turn to food to fill the void of separation from people.

I recommend the book *Getting Real* by Susan Campbell[10] as a primer for anyone wanting to improve communication skills. Her "Ten Truth Skills" practiced consistently are a great jump start to effective communication.

Managing the PDM—Reaction vs. Response

The third part of the empowerment shift for sabotage #3 is Managing the PDM (Protective Default Mechanism). When we react to situations or people with an automatic, fear-based PDM strategy, including overeating, our world stays contracted and small, without the possibility of inner peace. Our PDM also provokes PDMs in others, thus perpetuating the cycle. Our PDMs are automatic, predictable, and reactive. Stepping into our personal power requires that we stop the reactive tendencies and choose instead to respond with compassion and wisdom.

When we respond to those same situations or people from a love-based being of Essence, a whole new world opens up for us, as our perception of that world is now different. Our context shifts. We don't need the fear-based defensive strategies, because with compassion and wisdom we can choose different responses, including trust and effective communication.

When we practice shifting our PDM to Essence, our authentic self, our PDM begins to shrink in power and energy. It's as if we had a saber-toothed tiger with its jaws around our neck, dragging us down ... very scary. But when we distinguish what's going on, the tiger becomes a tiny Chihuahua, whose little bark is "Arf, Arf, Arf," not the menacing tiger's "Grrrrrrrrrrrowl."

So how do we shift from reactive PDM to responsive Essence? I love the concept of an "Essence Resource Guide," a term that I coined to represent a document, page, or file in which we list ways that we can bring ourselves back to Essence. The following are examples of Essence Resource Guide tools and activities, which some of my clients utilize:

- Distinguishing the PDM and the underlying fear
- Reminding yourself of your Essence
- Pausing
- Being curious instead of reactive
- Meditation or prayer
- Listening to favorite music
- Playing with pet
- Taking a walk
- Working out
- Dancing
- Calling a friend or your coach
- Writing in your journal
- Noticing where you are incomplete and doing a completion

- Exercise/activity
- Being in nature
- Getting a good night's sleep
- Providing or asking for acknowledgment
- Providing or asking for service
- Finding a different perspective (context)

Howard, my executive client, distinguished that his PDM of gruffness was based on his fear of not being a good enough leader and losing respect from his direct reports. He remembered that his Essence included Wisdom and Compassion. When he practiced leadership from Essence, he no longer needed a façade of gruffness to gain respect, his feelings of being a fraud evaporated, and his people began opening up with him, no longer feeling that they needed to protect themselves. As we worked together in our executive coaching sessions, Howard also dropped his excess weight.

How I Practiced Trust, Communication, and Managing My PDM with New In-Laws

In my new marriage we prepared to spend the holidays with his parents in another town. I was participating in a food plan (O.W.L. Level 1 Food Plan) which called for only whole foods without any grains. My new in-laws usually served food that was processed or made with ingredients that were not on my plan. They had very few vegetables, if any, on the menu and usually served an excess of starches, such as breads, potatoes, and desserts. They were unaware of the health or weight-gain risks that I wanted to change, and they certainly were unaware of my food addictions, especially to sugar and flour. As our travel date crept closer, I envisioned conversations with repeated explanations on my part and judgments on their part. I knew I would cave in with any confrontation. I was afraid to ask my husband for help because he didn't have a weight problem, and I didn't think he would understand either. I had no idea how I would navigate the holiday season and stick to my program with integrity. So I wanted to skip the trip altogether to protect myself from the expected discomfort and to avoid having to share my food addictions. My other alternative was to fall off the plan and eat everything and anything I wanted, thus putting myself out of integrity and opposing my commitment. Either of these choices avoided setting and keeping boundaries for myself.

I complained to my friends about my lack of willpower, my relatives' poor eating habits, and the whole situation! My Protection and Fear of Intimacy sabotage pattern was kicking in ... and kicking my butt! I then realized that I was not practicing what I preach. I was not trusting myself, my new relatives, or anything else. I also was not practicing empowered communication. I was coming from my Protective Default Mechanism. I had gone into the mode of victim, and I wanted to break this pattern.

So for my holiday "dilemma" I got back into being "at cause." I first made a choice to trust myself, my new family, and the circumstances. I chose to trust myself to set firm boundaries, and I chose to trust my husband to hear me and to validate me. I also chose to make two requests. The first was asking my husband to support me in setting my food boundaries with his family. The second request was to his family regarding the menu, what I needed, and how I could contribute. My decision to be proactive put me back into my Essence, and my holiday eating experience was successful!

Reason 4:
Playing Small

In your life a new day is dawning
Awaken and touch the beauty
Wherever you've come from
Whatever you've been
New possibilities beckon right here and now
Awaken and make them real
There was a time when you held in your heart
The most magnificent of dreams
A time when life seemed to carry
Endless promises and possibilities
Those dreams are still with you
Awaken and bring them to life
What you long for is longing for you
What you dream of is what you are meant to create
—Ralph S. Marston, Jr.

The Sabotage Pattern

*P*laying Small is a sabotage pattern that we consciously or unconsciously run that dampens our experience of life. It affects our ability to step into our full power and possibility. Our fears of not being "enough" or not being lovable keep us small. Our PDMs want us to stay in our comfort zone because stepping outside is perceived as dangerous by the PDM. So the strategy of the PDM is to Play Small, meaning play it easy, safe, comfortable, withdrawn, and/or lazy ... anything where people shrink from playing full-out and believing in their greatness. It comes from a context/perspective of "I don't matter" or "I'm not good enough" or "I'm not lovable."

When people don't think they matter, they fill their lives with time-wasters and fear-based activities. They hide out, or withdraw or play it safe. There is no passion for something bigger than themselves. They take the coward's way out. With regard to food and exercise, it doesn't matter anyway, so why be committed? It's easier to eat the junk food and to watch the boob tube or play electronic games. It's safer to not risk getting outside of the comfort zone or showing up.

The Playing Small sabotage doesn't always look like "lazy couch potato bum." It can show up when we don't speak up for ourselves, when we avoid confrontation, or when we acquiesce to keep the peace. It can show up when we withhold our opinions for fear of being pushy, meddlesome, nosy, or wrong. Playing Small can show up as a reticence to contribute, shying away from visibility, and a resistance to taking risks. The Playing Small sabotage pattern keeps us in same old, same old mode. We let our fears of the unknown be bigger than our commitment to playing full-out. The underlying context of "I'm not enough" keeps us from reaching for even higher standards of excellence or accomplishing our dreams and possibilities.

In working with clients in organizations and also with entrepreneurs, I often see the sabotage pattern of Playing Small emerge. In all levels of an organization, employees often hold back their opinions and ideas with the unconscious or conscious belief that it won't make a difference. I see this also in the realm of social change. People don't like how something is done, perhaps within government, but they do nothing about it, again believing that they can't make a difference. Entrepreneurs often play small in settling for smaller results, timid marketing efforts, undercharging, and undervaluing themselves and their services.

Isabel, a brilliant woman with a PhD, was an executive vice president for a research company. She hired me because she didn't understand why she was passed over for promotions and wanted to remedy that, and because she wanted to be less intimidated and more powerful in communicating with the company president. In our work, Isabel discovered how and when she played small at work, thus sabotaging her progress and confidence. When she let go of this sabotage, Isabel empowered herself and her communication, improved her relationship with her employees, and concurrently stopped her nightly eating/drinking regimen, which she had previously used as a coping/comfort strategy.

How are you playing small in your life? Is it in your marketing of your business? Is it in giving up on your dream career? Is it in fear of new experiences? Are you playing small in your health, your finances, your relationships, or your passions?

The problem with Playing Small arises because it is incongruous with who we really are, our magnificent Essential Self. Deep down we know that there is more. Deep down we know that the person we knew we could be is still waiting to be seen and heard. Deep down, consciously or subconsciously, we know that we have an unexpressed purpose that Playing Small does not allow to surface.

Our Deepest Fear

One of my favorite quotes is "Our Deepest Fear" from *A Return to Love* by Marianne Williamson.[11] This passage represents my belief about people and why I developed my mission to help people worldwide to love and accept themselves.

Our deepest fear is not that we are inadequate.
Our deepest fear is that we are powerful beyond measure.
It is our light, not our darkness that most frightens us.

We ask ourselves, "Who am I to be brilliant, gorgeous, talented, fabulous?"

*Actually, who are you not to be? You are a child of God.
Your playing small does not serve the world. There is
nothing enlightened about shrinking
so that other people won't feel insecure around you.*

*We are all meant to shine, as children do.
We were born to make manifest the glory
of God that is within us.
It is not just in some of us; it is in everyone.
And as we let our own light shine, we unconsciously give
other people permission to do the same.
As we are liberated from our own fear, our presence
automatically liberates others.*

How does the sabotage pattern of playing small affect our weight? We hold back from full enjoyment and fulfillment of life because of the fear—fear of being exposed as not enough or unlovable. Since holding back is out of alignment with our true essential nature and since we don't want to feel the fear, we suppress. We suppress with compulsions such as spending, drugs, alcohol, gambling, sex, or food. Thus, we suppress our magnificence.

A few years ago I realized how small I was playing when I spent much of my time behind the computer instead of networking, speaking, and marketing myself. I was afraid of exposure and rejection. Ready for a breakthrough in this area, I hired coach/mentor Kailash Sozzani for a total makeover, which exponentially raised my confidence and changed the way I see myself. Kailash's loving attention helped to transform me from the outside in. Next I hired Zimmerman Photography Studio to integrate my Kailash makeover with my marketing. Experts Kyle, Max, and Kate highlighted a perspective of me that I didn't think existed: beauty and grace. Through their professional photos, videos, and social media assistance, I began to really believe that I could stop playing small and gain professional credibility and visibility.

But just looking the part doesn't fix playing small. We must look deeper to our Big, Big Why—Our Life Purpose.

What to Do About It: Alignment with Purpose

Shifting from Playing Small requires two things: Courage and Alignment with Purpose. Courage simply means having the capacity (ability to embrace courage) and willingness to change. Courage is a decision. Courage comes from within.

Alignment with Purpose means distinguishing our life purpose and committing to it on a daily basis. Many books, seminars, and workshops address finding your life purpose. The simplest description I have found comes from *A New Earth: Awakening to Your Life's Purpose* by Eckhart Tolle.[12] Tolle maintains that our inner, primary purpose is to be in the present moment. In Ontological Weight Loss terminology, our purpose is to be in our Essence—our authentic Being— every moment. When we practice and improve our capacity to be in the present moment, Tolle says we have a secondary or outer purpose, which is the doing. Our secondary purpose is what we do and how we take our talents and gifts to the world.

Primary and Secondary Purpose

If your inner, primary purpose is your essence, what is your secondary purpose, your outer, doing purpose? The easiest way to uncover your secondary purpose is to reflect on what comes easily and naturally for you. What do you love to do? What do others think is hard, yet you think is easy? For example, do you like to cheer people up? Or do you really love people? Do you love to teach people things? Are you a natural leader? Are you automatically compassionate? Do you love to empower others? Write down several things that you know you do automatically and predictably and that you love when you are doing them. Now look at those words and get the sense of them, the common themes. You are getting closer to your life purpose. What is a phrase that captures your heart?

The following examples of life purpose have been provided from selected clients:

- I Shift the Planet
- Goddess of Empowerment
- Breath of Life
- Breath of Love
- Facilitator
- Sage
- Inspiration
- Heaven on Earth
- Goddess of Possibility
- Angel
- Creating Joy
- Divine Inspiration

Your purpose doesn't have to mimic these, and I trust you understand the concept. Your purpose is your gift to the world. Being on purpose every day is how you stay fulfilled. Being on purpose every day is how you transform the Playing Small sabotage. And that translates to health and weight maintenance because you no longer have to turn to food or withhold yourself in order to fill the deeper, grander longing of what we're all about.

My weight-loss client, Jerri, had difficulty sticking with her Lifetime Level 4 food plan. She had dropped 50 pounds in her Private Platinum O.W.L. Program with me, but during her final phase, old habits began to return. Jerri thought her sabotage was Sacrifice and Entitlement, because she would binge and then feel guilty. But I asked her to consider that the Playing Small sabotage pattern kept her stuck. She only binged to compensate for not being and doing what really lit her up in life. The off-program food represented a substitute for the excitement and purpose that called her (and that she ignored). Once Jerri considered a shift from Playing Small to Alignment with Purpose, her day-to-day life took on new meaning, and her food did too.

Our life purpose helps us know how to give our gifts to the world. A schoolteacher aligns her purpose of "I shift the planet" with her career. A public speaker aligns his purpose of "Divine Inspiration" with his career.

I struggled for many years to identify and understand my purpose in life. I knew I loved to help people love and believe in themselves, because I did that naturally and automatically. But I didn't know how it related to a life purpose. Although they were not aware of their impact, two people helped me clarify my purpose.

The first was my dear friend, Nancy Parkhill, who died of cancer in 2003. As I supported her during her death process, Nancy often talked about what she had done with her life and what she wished she had done. She spoke of dreams and regrets. After her passing, I asked myself these and similar questions: "When I am on my deathbed, what will I know that I have done with my life?" "What am I here to do?" "What is my purpose on this planet?" Answers came spontaneously (unprompted) through three unrelated people who volunteered their advice that I should be a life coach. Shortly thereafter, I enrolled in a comprehensive coach training program and began a new career as an ontological/facilitative life and business coach. I knew at a deep level that an ontological coaching career was in alignment with my purpose. Even without descriptive words, I could feel the resonance. I no longer needed to cling to past roles of CPA or Mary Kay Senior Sales Director, which had become unfulfilling.

Further guiding me toward my life purpose was my mentor, Hans Phillips, who co-founded my first coach training program. Hans taught me to let go of self-criticism, playing small, and cynicism, so that I could step into a position of leadership and serving others worldwide. Hans brought a small rubber ball in the shape of a globe to our training classes. At random he would throw the ball toward someone unexpectedly during class with these words: "Here's the world. It's in your hands. What are you going to do with it?" His metaphor and symbol helped me to see how each of us can make a global impact, whether we know it or not.

Thanks to Nancy and Hans, I shifted my Playing Small sabotage pattern to Alignment with Purpose. In my previous careers as a CPA and as a Mary Kay senior sales director, my favorite activities were helping people feel better about themselves and their businesses, not the tax laws or the cosmetics. I learned that I am aligned with purpose when I take my primary purpose of being my essence (Joy, Compassion, Serenity, Leadership, Courage, and Grace) into the world by inspiring people to identify, uncover, and become their best, next version of themselves. I adopted "I am the breath of love and life" as my life purpose statement.

When I am being and acting in alignment with my purpose, I choose to stay fit and healthy so that I maintain the energy and vitality to remain impassioned and productive in creating my grand mission. I also want to be a good role model for my clients. Do you know there is something more for you? Are you bored or confused with where you are? Do you have a mission and a vision greater than your PDM? If so, do you read it daily and does it inspire you? If not, why not? Are you "playing small"? Are you ready to create your vision and mission for your life so that you can step into the next higher version of you?

Identifying and pursuing a fulfilling life and career begins with knowing your own purpose. Once you have a sense of your purpose, you may begin to notice where you are in alignment with it and where you are not. The first time I met my husband Jay, I asked him to tell me about himself. He answered, "Who I am is not what I do." Wow! He was definitely NOT in alignment with his purpose. His schooling and his love were in psychology, but in college he fell into construction as a way to pay bills. He stayed with construction, but his heart was not in it. Jay's secondary purpose was to help others align with their full magnificence and spirit through some kind of counseling support. Recently, Jay completed training and certification to be a licensed hypnotherapist. When he transitioned from construction contractor to hypnotherapist, Jay became aligned with his purpose of helping others.

You may experience consequences when aligning with your purpose: discomfort and resistance for you, not to mention discomfort and resistance from others, especially if it means others have to change something—usually their perspective. When my granddaughter graduated from high school as "straight A" valedictorian, she received a full scholarship to attend the school of her choice in the state. But she dropped out of college within a couple of weeks after registration in order to explore a different pathway, one in which she felt that she was following her purpose. Her mother and I were disappointed, maybe even devastated, and had to adjust our perspective on her choice. But she had the courage to choose what was right for herself at the time and continues to do so now.

When Jay began turning down construction jobs as he transitioned to a hypnotherapy business, his longtime customers, who counted on his expertise and reliability, had to adjust their perspective on what Jay "should" be doing.

When I transitioned from a career as a CPA to helping people build successful home businesses in Mary Kay Cosmetics, my family disapproved. They asked, "Why did you spend all that time and money getting your master's degree and taking the CPA exam just to sell lipsticks?" They didn't realize that my passion and purpose was to inspire and uplift others. They didn't realize that tax laws were not in alignment with that purpose.

How do you want to be remembered? When you are celebrating your 100th birthday or are on your deathbed, what do you want remembered about yourself and what you accomplished or contributed? What fulfilled you? This reflection helps you determine your purpose. And the same reflection helps you determine your business purpose. With that mindset, you might also wish to write your vision and mission statement for your life and for your career.

I've come to believe that each of us has a personal calling that's as unique as a fingerprint—and that the best way to succeed is to discover what you love and then find a way to offer it to others in the form of service, working hard, and also allowing the energy of the universe to lead you.
—Oprah Winfrey

Reason 5:
Incompletion

The health of your body influences what
you experience in your mind.
There is no split.
If you can engage your whole spirit
in the pursuit of total fitness
—not just your intellect, not just your emotions—
but instead everything inside you that is truly you,
you'll discover what it is to be a whole person.
—David Patchell-Evans

The Sabotage Pattern

Incompletion is a major sabotage pattern, which includes mental and emotional energy drains, ranging from simple things such as unfinished work tasks to more complex things such as unresolved issues from the past, unfinished emotional business, or communication issues. To clarify, incompletion includes more than being unfinished; it addresses the mental, emotional, or energetic drain that we perceive.

In contrast, completion aids us in letting go of the source of any energy drain or attention drain and, therefore, empowers us. Completion is the opportunity to be present, to release energy drains, to be acknowledged, and to celebrate. We may not necessarily be finished, per se, but we are energetically complete and ready for what is next. Completion empowers us in terms of freeing up time, attention, focus, energy, power, and essence. We often resist and fear completion because completion disturbs our Protective Default Mechanism's sense of balance. The PDM's purpose is to protect you, so it looks for something from which to protect you. Therefore, if you are incomplete with something in the past, the PDM gets to "protect you" with a fear-based strategy, such as anger, defensiveness, regret, or depression. All PDM strategies rob you of your full power and energy. Unwillingness to be complete is a sign of a victim context, whereby we remain "at the effect" of someone, something, or some circumstance. Incompletion exhausts you with the unproductive energy it consumes. To compensate, we try to boost our energy in other ways. If you notice you are sleeping a lot, consuming unhealthy foods or beverages, or engaging in other compulsive/addictive activities, you may be resisting completion in one or more areas of your life.

Incompletion can arise in any area, such as the end of a project, a graduation, a mistake, an argument, selling a home, relationship changes, or the ending or change of a career. For example, at the end of the day, do you berate yourself for not getting all your tasks done? When you make a mistake, do you worry and fret? When a relationship ends, do you rehash what happened countless times? When you have an argument, do you stew and blame? When you change residences, do you stuff down emotions about it? Any time you are incomplete in any area, you sabotage yourself energetically and emotionally.

Karina did not hire me for her weight loss but because she was angry all the time and wanted to regain her peace of mind. Through coaching Karina uncovered a deep resentment (incompletion) toward her ex-husband for his unfaithfulness and financial irresponsibility while they were married. She carried a grudge around like a weight around her neck. It was no coincidence that she also carried 30 extra pounds. In the coaching work that we did together, Karina released the negative energy that weighed her down. She regained her peace of mind and dropped her excess weight.

What to Do About It: Completion, Compassion, and Forgiveness

The empowerment pattern from the sabotage pattern of Incompletion includes Completion, Compassion, and Forgiveness. Completion doesn't necessarily mean "finished." Completion is any energetic release. It includes saying what needs to be said and then setting an intention and making a declaration to be complete. If I have an argument with my husband, I may choose to harbor hurt and anger, or I may choose to get "complete." Perhaps I would apologize. Perhaps I would ask him for an apology. Perhaps I would realize I was being overly dramatic and just choose to let it go. Regardless of whichever way I get complete, I release any negative energy that I am carrying.

Ultimately upon being complete, we will probably embrace acceptance, and even forgiveness or celebration. Afterward, the event carries the same energy as last month's breakfast. We know it happened, but it's over. How do we become complete? There is no right or wrong way to become complete. The first step is willingness, and the second step is to choose a manner of completion.

Completion may be as simple as shutting a door that is open or tying a shoe that is untied. It may be scheduling a time to finish a project. It may be having a conversation with someone or journaling. If anger is involved, completion may be facilitated by doing something physical to get the emotion released from your body.

I'll share a variety of the methods I recommend to be complete. Which of the following completion methods have you tried or would you be willing to try?

- Schedule time to finish a project and do it. Acknowledge yourself when done.
- Schedule a time for a celebration and celebrate.

- Physical/emotional release: Pound on a pillow, scream, work out, go for a long hike or run, punch a punching bag, etc.
- Visualize yourself complete, releasing any negative energies, and forgiving yourself and/or the other person.
- Simple declaration and release: "I refuse to let this bother me anymore; I declare myself to be complete."

Resentment

Resentment is the number-one offender in the area of incompletion. Resentment causes trouble because it triggers overeating and other compulsions when we stuff or suppress the emotions arising from incompletion. Resentment is an area where we often are not willing to be complete, because we think if we become complete via forgiveness or compassion, it means we have given our personal power away to that person. There are consequences of forgiveness, including giving up resentment, anger, defensiveness. Our PDM doesn't want to give up these if we see them as our only means to power. But if we don't get complete, we're basically vomiting our past into our future. When we complete and let go of resentments, choosing compassion and forgiveness instead, we actually empower ourselves.

Leah carried the burden of anger and resentment toward her husband of 20 years. In her perception, he was consumed with career and self to the point that she did not feel respected, supported, or cherished. When I introduced the topic of completion and how she gave her power away, she realized that she was not willing to give up her PDM of anger and resentment, since she thought it represented strength and power. Through coaching, she learned that her strength and power included more effective tools, such as empowered communication, boundaries, and belief in herself.

Maybe your resentments are toward yourself and you need to forgive yourself in order to be complete. Regardless, the process is the same and includes responsibility, mercy, listening deeply, compassion, and grace in order to become complete. In the process of becoming complete, there is the decision to release the emotional hold of the incompletion. In doing so, there is healing, allowing, forgiveness, and acceptance, thus freeing up the energy to move forward to what's next.

I suggest you begin by practicing completion everywhere. For more emotional triggers, resentments, and so on, consider hiring an ontological coach or a therapist if you are unable or unwilling to become complete.

Reason 6:
Addiction To Suffering

May today there be peace within. May you trust
that you are exactly where you are meant to be. May you
not forget the infinite possibilities that are born of faith in
yourself and others. May you use the gifts that you have
received, and pass on the love that has been given to you.
May you be content with yourself just the way you are.
Let this knowledge settle into your bones, and allow your
soul the freedom to sing, dance, praise and love.
It is there for each and every one of us.
—Saint Terese of Liseaux

The Sabotage Pattern

The next unconscious sabotage pattern is pervasive, cunning, and ubiquitous: Addiction to Suffering. The unwillingness to be complete or to let go of resentment, as we discussed in the previous sabotage pattern, is one sign of Addiction to Suffering. Other signs include hopelessness and resignation. The pattern of Addiction to Suffering often manifests itself as quitting, forcing, or staying stuck. When you give up on yourself, such as quitting your weight-loss program, you are running the sabotage of Addiction to Suffering. When you go into pity parties, blame others, or blame circumstances, you have consciously or unconsciously engaged the Addiction to Suffering sabotage pattern. Another sign is feeling "stuck between a rock and a hard place."

These thoughts or words indicate your Addiction to Suffering sabotage pattern is active:

- I can't stick to my program
- My friends told me to just eat it this one time
- It won't matter anyway, because I'm always going to be fat
- Nothing works
- I've tried everything
- You can't make me
- I give up
- I want what I want when I want it; then I feel guilty … It's a vicious circle
- I hate my body, but there's nothing I can do about it
- Complaints without proactivity (requests or demands)
- Feeling stuck and resigned

Just as in the Incompletion sabotage, the context for Addiction to Suffering is the victim context, the perspective of being "at the effect" of something or someone, rather than at cause. When we consider how we are at cause for our resentments, for instance, we shift a victim context to a responsible context—that of being "at cause."

Marie's weight frustrated and angered her. She tried many diets without lasting success, ultimately deciding that nothing would work, and resigned herself to be overweight forever. But she was not "complete" energetically with this decision. She criticized herself every time she looked in the mirror or dressed. Intimacy with her husband suffered. She made excuses to herself and to her friends, including heredity, stress, metabolism, the environment and work and home, and willpower. The Addiction to Suffering sabotage was well entrenched in Marie's psyche.

What to Do About It: CHOICE—in Context, Belief, Vision, Possibility, and Commitment

A context of being "at cause" allows you to shift from the Addiction to Suffering sabotage pattern to an effective and productive mindset in your weight-loss journey. The overall theme in the shift can be described as Choice, which involves choosing your Context, your Belief, your Vision, your Possibility, and your Commitment. Let's explore each of these.

- Choosing Context: Declaring a context of "I get to choose" is the first step. If you don't believe that you get to choose, you must change that belief and choose another one.
- Choosing Belief: Do you believe that you get to choose and that you can have what you choose? Belief is a choice; it is not an inherited, genetic body part like blue eyes. It doesn't have to automatically be whatever you thought you believed. You get to choose your beliefs. What distinguishes winners in any area of life is their belief that they can be a winner, regardless of outside circumstances or other people's beliefs about them. What do you choose to believe? Does that belief empower you, make you a better person, and bring you peace?
- Choosing Vision: Many of my weight-loss clients, especially those who have always been overweight or have been overweight for a very long time, experience difficulty articulating or even imagining a vision of themselves at their ideal weight. Unconsciously, they believe that their past equals their future. However, the past does not equal the future, and we can imagine and create a vision of our choosing.

Neil had been overweight his whole life and could not imagine any other scenario. To access an inspiring vision for himself, I asked Neil to first list what he hated about being overweight and then to write the opposite. This writing with our coaching helped him create a motivating vision. What vision will you choose to inspire yourself?

> *If you can imagine it, you can achieve it.*
> *If you can dream it, you can become it.*
> —William Arthur Ward

- Choosing Possibility: In a self-development course years ago I learned this distinction. When you have an expectation that doesn't get met, the result is disappointment. When you have a possibility that doesn't get met, the result is still possibility. Possibility never dies. What is your possibility? Is your possibility to be healthy, fit, and strong? Is your possibility to be at your ideal weight, look good in your clothes, and be proud of your body? What possibility do you choose? Instead of expectation and disappointment, choose a possibility that propels you forward, regardless of the circumstances.

- Choosing Commitment: Many overweight people have conflicting or competing commitments. For example, my clients often say they are committed to dropping weight, but we then discover that they are also committed to a sabotage of Entitlement—"I get to eat whatever I want." They are committed to dropping weight, but then we discover that they are also committed to the comfort of being a couch potato. When our commitments conflict with each other, our progress is inconsistent or halts altogether. But most of us haven't yet made the first distinction that we have unconscious commitments nor the second distinction that those unconscious commitments compete or conflict with other commitments. What are your REAL commitments? Do they conflict or compete with each other? From a context of choice, belief, vision, and possibility, what commitment do you choose?

Until one is committed, there is hesitancy, the chance to draw back, always ineffectiveness. Concerning all acts of initiative (and creation), there is one elementary truth, the ignorance of which kills countless ideas and splendid plans: that the moment one definitely commits oneself, then Providence moves too. All sorts of things occur to help one that would never otherwise have occurred. A whole stream of events issue from the decision, raising in one's favour all manner of unforeseen incidents and meetings and material assistance, which no man could have dreamed would have come his way. I have learned a deep respect for one of Goethe's couplets:

Whatever you can do, or dream you can, begin it.
Boldness has genius, power, and magic in it.

—W. H. Murray, *The Scottish Himalayan Expedition*

When you don't have a vision, don't see the possibility, and don't remember your commitment, you revert to the Addiction to Suffering sabotage and slide back into yo-yo dieting and the other sabotages. When the vision is clear and compelling, it propels us forward. Your job is to keep the context of choice alive.

What if every time you noticed you were suffering, you decided that you refuse to suffer anymore? What would change for you? What would take the place of the suffering? What would you do differently?

On which vision for success would you like to focus every day? Does it inspire you and pull you forward?

What are all of your commitments in the area of weight loss? Do they support and enhance each other, or do they compete or conflict with each other? If they conflict, how will you prioritize them?

Reason 7:
Separate, Alone, And Hard

There can be no vulnerability without risk; there can be no community without vulnerability; there can be no peace, and ultimately no life, without community.
—M. Scott Peck

The Sabotage Pattern

*D*id you know that weight-loss success, especially long-term success, correlates with receiving and giving support? People who are in a group, have a buddy, and are accountable to someone else reach their goals faster and keep weight off longer. (This is one reason we created the "Keep It Off Club.")

However, a vast majority of overweight people do not receive the kind of support that they need. Since how we do one thing is how we do everything, not being supported shows up in other areas too. In sabotage #2 we learned that Well-Being is a pillar of success, yet so many overweight people put others' needs before their own needs. In sabotage #3 we learned that Protection and Fear of Intimacy keep us defended. The belief of "I'm not good enough" or "I'm not deserving" underlies those and is reflected in a similar way here with sabotage #7. It looks like "I must prove that I am good enough, so I will do it all myself" or "I don't deserve to receive help."

A sense of unworthiness or embarrassment restricts us in admitting that we need help or in asking for it. When we reach out to others, we run the risk of vulnerability and open ourselves to perceived criticism, usually because we are already criticizing ourselves. Or we don't want to risk looking bad or give up looking good because that would be embarrassing and confronting. It would confirm our deepest fear—that we are not enough. So it's easier not to open up or request support.

Earlier in my coaching career, I resisted asking for help from my mastery advanced coaching group, my coach, or on a mastermind support call. If I shared my breakdowns, I wouldn't look like I had it all together. I would also look like the hot mess I saw myself being, and that would be risky. What if they disrespected me for it? What if they judged me and thought I was a weak coach? In holding back from asking and receiving support, I was playing the game of Separate, Alone, and Hard.

There are other risks of connecting, sharing, and requesting support, including exposure to other people's fear-based Protective Default Mechanisms, in addition to our own. When I was a newlywed, I learned quickly that if I shared that I was worried about something, such as having enough money to pay bills, my husband thought I was criticizing him for not earning enough, even though I was not criticizing, just sharing my worry. My protective default patterns provoked his. As a leader, I have worried that if I show my weaknesses, my followers will have doubt and worries too. A person who feels responsible for others may not connect totally for fear of affecting them negatively.

In one of my O.W.L. Weight Loss groups, Missy did not report her slips or binges with her food program for fear of being a bad influence on the rest of the group. She wanted to "look good" and to be a shining example for everyone, but that noble cause hurt her own progress.

Mel, my own accountability buddy, never told me she was eating chocolate on the sly because she didn't want me to quit my own program. However, this separate and alone sabotage cost her the opportunity to get the support she needed regarding her chocolate binges.

These two examples represent a form of codependency, sabotaging our own authentic progress to take care of someone else.

People who are overweight or are in debt or in any compulsion are usually carrying secrets around that are too embarrassing for them to share. They associate guilt and shame with their actions, such as falling off their plan or having cravings. This often shows up in our "Keep It Off Club," a membership group of people who want to continue and maintain their weight-loss successes via online support, bimonthly training, and Q&A calls. When I coach weight-loss clients and ask them to post their progress on the "Keep It Off Club" online forum, it can be very confronting for them. Some will learn that there isn't anything to fear and that the group is friendly and supportive. Others will never share anything that goes wrong; they just share good stuff. Some find it is a great resource. Some discover that sharing is a way to empower themselves by having connection and relationship with people who are on the same page.

Margaret, a graduate of the six-month O.W.L. Private Platinum Weight Loss Program, confessed that her least favorite part of the program was posting her progress and accountabilities on the "Keep It Off Club." She said, actually, that she hated it at first! When I asked her which parts of the program contributed most significantly to her success, one of her answers was, predictably, posting on the "Keep It Off Club." She had transformed "Separate, Alone, and Hard" to the empowerment shift and dropped 50 pounds in the process. Even after reaching her goal weight, Margaret continues as a member of the "Keep It Off Club" and posts daily.

Sometimes it never occurs to us to ask for help. Often we've been doing it ourselves for so long that we don't even think about asking for help. This is an example of an unconscious sabotage.

Or maybe our PDMs don't want to give up control, so we resist asking for help because we think we can do it better or faster without a helper. If we are operating under a fear-based need to control or avoid being controlled, the opportunity for relating and connecting is diminished and so is the opportunity to stop the sabotage pattern.

Maybe we have a subconscious need to prove our worth to others, or to ourselves. Whatever the reason—conscious or not—the mindset of having to do it all, feeling alone, and separating ourselves from others makes things harder. We isolate ourselves from resources that could make thing easier for us.

Do you separate yourself from others? Do you power through projects and challenges alone? Do you resist sharing and connecting? Do you hold back feelings and emotions due to embarrassment or fear of looking bad or wanting to be in control? Do you do all the work yourself instead of asking for help? These are some of the signs of running "Separate, Alone, and Hard" sabotage #7. Also remember, if you do this in any other area of your life, you are probably doing it in your weight-loss efforts.

What to Do About It: Connection, Partnering, and Support

When we vulnerably step out of the realm of going solo and into the empowerment shift to Connection, Partnering, and Support, we access and express courage and strength. It's a sign of a strong character and a role model for the rest of us. The transparency and authenticity required for this shift inspire others to do the same. My mentor Hans once told me, "Janis, when you share yourself, you are an inspiration, even in your breakdowns, and especially in your breakdowns."

Another benefit of this shift includes the gift of other people's Essence. Their love, wisdom, and experience are valuable resources. When we are willing to request and discover support, we open up possibility for it to give us exactly what we need. Connection, Partnering, and Support with others as resources speeds up, simplifies, and uplifts.

When I was a CPA, I remember struggling for hours to understand a client's financial scribbled notes because I was too embarrassed to call him. I didn't want to look stupid. Later in life I learned that if I make a call or send an email immediately when I am stuck, I get answers quickly and move forward. (And instead of looking stupid, I appear efficient.)

When I crave a food not on my plan and struggle with my willpower, talking myself in and out of eating it over and over, the results may be that I give up or give in. However, when I pick up the phone and call my buddy or send an email to my group, I have the opportunity to shift the craving with awareness, understanding, compassion, and a different set of choices that come with connection, partnering, and support. This involves NO struggle—only willingness to open up and share myself with others.

> *If you have one idea and I have one idea, we each have an idea. But if you share your idea with me and I share mine with you, we each have two ideas.*
> —Author unknown; taught by Mary Kay Ash

If I get sloppy with my commitment to go to the gym, I can talk myself out of it in a heartbeat with any excuse. If you need an excuse, any one will do! But when I ask for support with an accountability buddy or a workout partner, I am less likely to bail on myself and more likely to have fun.

My clients, like Margaret, who share themselves regularly and consistently on the "Keep It Off Club" and with their weight-loss buddies are much more successful long term than those who don't.

My own belief and behavior pattern told me that I had to do things myself. I was stuck in the Separate, Alone, and Hard sabotage. I have been blessed with several coaches and mentors through the years who helped me distinguish this and learn that I could shift the pattern.

Although difficult at first, I learned that there is no shame in asking others for support. As a matter of fact, it inspires others to do the same, reducing the time and energy of being stuck.

A significant empowerment shift from Separate, Alone, and Hard to Connection, Partnering, and Support occurred during my two-year participation in Ontological Master Mind (O.M.M.), a group of amazing coaches, including Salley Trefethen, Anna Meck, Leslie

Carleton, and Pamela Catey. I really didn't want to participate at first, since it seemed a waste of time, when I had "so much to do." But I realized the power of masterminding and agreed. We all graduated from the Accomplishment Coaching Coach Training and Leadership Program and lived in the same city, so we banded together in pursuit of inspiration for our coaching specialties. Through mutual support and brainstorming, the concept for my baby was born—Ontological Weight Loss (O.W.L.): Your Once-in-a-Lifetime Solution. The empowerment pattern of Connection, Partnering, and Support had resulted in a major shift in the direction of my coaching business.

After O.M.M. was over, I later worked with Pamela for marketing coaching and inner work coaching. One of the many valuable lessons Pamela reflected back to me was my ability to utilize the skills and resources I already have instead of needing to create new ones. That alone was worth the price of admission, as I shifted Hard to Easy. Pamela was also instrumental in supporting me and dissolving my intense fear of marketing.

The creation of the O. W. L. Weight Loss Program name is another example of my breakthrough to an empowerment pattern of Connection, Partnering, and Support. When I searched for a tagline to Ontological Weight Loss, my coach Jamie Sue Johnson inspired the subtitle: "Your Once-in-a-Lifetime Solution." Wow! That was easy!

We are all angels with one wing.
It is only when we hold hands that we can fly.
—Taught by Mary Kay Ash

In addition to connecting, partnering, and support with other people, this empowerment shift includes an alliance and relationship with the whole Divinity Triangle: Others, yourself in the form of wisdom and intuition, and the Divine (God, the Universe, Spirit). The practice of giving trust as a gift will help you shift sabotage #7.

So what do you need to create this transformation from Separate, Alone, and Hard to Connection, Partnering, and Support? Not much … just willingness, courage, and vulnerability. When you choose to practice the new empowerment pattern, your life and your weight-loss project become easier, in the flow, and a lot more fun.

Who is on your list of supporters in your weight-loss journey? What support could you request from each one; for example, your workout partner, accountability buddy, cheerleader, or celebration partner? Will you practice asking for help if you start to waver in your program? If you would not make a support request, what would you have to let go of in order to do so?

Creating partnership everywhere provides you with the ability to make your life easier. What would it take for you to improve your relationship with yourself? How about improving your relationship with others? What would it take for you to improve your relationship with God/Divine/Spirit/Universe (your word for this)?

Reason 8:
Self-Deprecation

*I must learn to love the fool in me—the one who feels
too much, talks too much, takes too many chances, wins
sometimes and loses often, lacks self-control, loves and hates,
hurts and gets hurt, promises and breaks promises,
laughs and cries. It alone protects me against that
utterly self-controlled, masterful tyrant whom
I also harbor and who would rob me of my human
aliveness, humility, and dignity but for my Fool.*
—Theodore I. Rubin

The Sabotage Pattern

Self-Deprecation, which means self-criticism, putting yourself down, or beating yourself up, is based on the unconscious context of "I'm not enough." Whenever you say disempowering things about yourself or are judgmental or critical, this is self-deprecation. This sabotage pattern, like all the rest of them, started early in your life. As a child you may have heard derogatory comments about yourself or about others, and for you they became normal. You may be using negativity unconsciously as a Protective Default Mechanism. The unconscious mindset of the PDM is, "If I criticize myself first, then no one else can criticize me."

Self-deprecation shows up in our relationship to ourselves, our bodies, and our actions. It reinforces the belief of "not enough" and adds to the feelings of unworthiness. It's a vicious, downward cycle: the unworthiness/not enough context evokes the self-criticism, and the self-criticism validates the feelings of unworthiness.

Self-deprecation is so prevalent. How many times have you received a compliment from someone and instead of allowing it to soak in, you diminished it with a "Thank you, but ..." either inwardly or out loud? Do you understate your brilliance? Do you withhold acknowledgment from yourself for big or small victories? Do you call yourself names? Are your accomplishments never good enough for you? Do you criticize yourself either explicitly or with your internal self-talk? Are you always saying, "I should have ..." to yourself? These are examples of self-deprecation.

When I notice my clients using the sabotage pattern of Self-Deprecation, such as believing the worst instead of the best about themselves, I call them out and ask them to rephrase the sentence. I ask them to practice noticing when they are doing it. I also ask them to hand over the big stick they are beating themselves up with.

Will, a very witty client, said to me once when I asked him to hand over the big stick, "It won't make a difference, Janis. I can order more of those big sticks on the Internet any time I want, and they come right to my door."

How this sabotage relates to weight is similar to the other sabotages: when we criticize ourselves we feel terrible about ourselves, so we compensate by trying to feel better, and our feel-good default is overeating or zoning out in some other way.

What to Do About It: Celebration, Gratitude, and Service

Shifting from the sabotage of Self-Deprecation involves the practices we discussed previously, such as noticing and rephrasing your wording. Words are very powerful in changing context (mindset) and beliefs about ourselves. In addition, the context shift includes returning to Essence, since Self-Deprecation clearly indicates a Protective Default

Mechanism pattern, stemming from the fear that "I'm not enough" or "I'm not good enough."

Returning to Your Essential Being: Your Essence Resource Guide

Since Self-Deprecation, like all sabotage patterns, comes from the Protective Default Mechanism, when we step from PDM into Essence, we have automatically dissolved the sabotage. We view ourselves with wisdom and love, not with fear. In the midst of a raging PDM, we don't always remember what Essence looks like or how to return to it. Creating an Essence Resource Guide, in which we include the many ways we can shift to Essence, is a great tool for remembering how to step into Essence when PDM pops out. It can happen in the blink of an eye! If you haven't already created an Essence Resource Guide, please do so now. If you did create one, this is a great time to review and revise it.

Your Essence Resource Guide should be created when you are already in your Essence and will include all the ways that you know help you to be there. Here are some of my own Essence Resource Guide ideas:

- Distinguish what's missing in my well-being and do one thing to close that gap. (I address physical, mental, emotional, spiritual, and other areas.)
- Distinguish where I am incomplete or out of integrity with myself or others; then I take action to get back into integrity.
- Do a completion exercise.
- Talk to a friend.
- Talk to my coach.
- Listen to music.
- Write in a journal.

- Get into my body with movement (walk, run, dance, work out, etc.).
- Pray or meditate.
- List my blessings—what I am grateful for.
- Spend time in nature.
- Read my Essence words to remember who I really am.
- Read my PDM words and ask myself, "What am I afraid of?" and "What do I need right now?" Then I take action on those answers to fulfill those needs and dissolve those fears.
- Read my Life Purpose.
- Read my vision.
- Ask myself these three questions,
  - "What is so (facts only)?"
  - "What is missing (disempowering, incomplete)?"
  - "What is next?"
- Ask myself, "Is this a fact or an interpretation?" (Most everything is interpretation unless it can be measured.)

What are more ways that you know you always return to Essence? I suggest adding those ideas to your Essence Resource Guide and reviewing it frequently. In addition to the list above, Celebration, Gratitude, and Service are excellent ways to return and stay in Essence. Let's understand each of those and why they shift the Self-Deprecation sabotage pattern.

Celebration

The more you praise and celebrate your life,
the more there is in life to celebrate.
—Oprah Winfrey

When we celebrate and acknowledge ourselves for what we do right, we no longer focus so dramatically on what we did wrong. We build the ontological muscle of seeing more of the good things and less of the bad for ourselves.

In my coaching sessions and the coaching preparation form, I always begin by asking my clients to share their wins, big or small. Many, if not most, of my clients have a difficult time with this in the beginning and even later in the coaching program. They are so used to looking at what is unfinished or missing that they can't name a single win. When I reflect back to them their victories which I see, they usually either discount them or declare they never thought of them as victories or anything to be acknowledged. They say things like, "That's not really a win. I do that every day." Or they say, "That's not a victory. I have to do it, so I do."

So I ask my clients, "What's up with that? Are you as stingy with your praise of others as you are with yourself? How about being a little more generous?" Often they resist, saying they don't think they or their actions deserve to be celebrated. Or they can't think of any ways to celebrate that they don't do already for themselves. Or they forget, another sign of resistance.

As an example, let's say you go off your food program, and the Self-Deprecation sabotage makes you really angry and harsh with yourself. Then you feel even worse. So you try to feel better by self-medicating, having more of the wrong foods, and saying, "I screwed up, so I just can't do it." Self-Deprecation and Addiction to Suffering are partners here. On the other hand, if you celebrate and acknowledge yourself, or if you ask your partner or friend or spouse to acknowledge you for all the times you stayed on your program and ate the right foods, you would tend to do more of that consistently. What you focus on expands. So you would look for more of those positive reinforcements and look forward to more celebrations and acknowledgments.

I am a stickler for teaching this concept, because celebration adds velocity—speed and power—to our weight-loss results by providing joy and anticipation. We accomplish our results faster. My new clients almost always resist acknowledging (praising) themselves at the end of our sessions. They haven't learned the importance of celebrating themselves. Praising ourselves is not being conceited; it's being smart and effective on a deeper level.

Celebration occurs on three levels:

- **Acknowledgment:** We RECOGNIZE AND DISTINGUISH an accomplishment, win, victory, effort, or progress—big or small.
- **Attitude:** We adopt an ATTITUDE or SPIRIT of joy and celebration, rather than diminishing the effort.
- **Reward:** We choose a TANGIBLE PRIZE for what we are acknowledging and celebrating. This can be something we already do or give ourselves, but we must correlate it to what we are celebrating and acknowledging.

Celebration should be consistent with the accomplishment. For smaller results or actions, we choose a small celebration. For medium-sized results or actions, we choose a medium celebration. And accordingly, for large results or actions, we choose a large celebration.

The following are examples of small, medium, and large accomplishments and their consistent rewards:

Small: You promised yourself that you would stick to your food plan for the whole day, and you did that. This was not hard, so you declare it to be a small accomplishment and reward. You email your coach to tell her, and then do a happy dance while shouting, "Woo hoo, I rock!"

Medium: You dropped five more pounds since you weighed in last month. This took some doing on your part, and you have 45 pounds to go. You declare that this is a medium accomplishment and celebration. You call your friend and schedule a play date to go shopping for a new scarf as your reward ... or you give yourself a day off from work ... or you schedule a massage and pedicure.

Large: You met your goal weight after dropping 50 pounds. This was a very big deal, a large accomplishment, and deserving of a large celebration. You schedule a week at a spa ... or you purchase a new outfit ... or you purchase a new wardrobe with the money you have been saving for this.

When we acknowledge, celebrate, and reward ourselves, we become motivated and excited to make more progress, because ontologically we have rewarded the preferred actions, not dwelled upon our mistakes.

Picture a little child with a messy room. You say, "If you clean up your room, we will go to the zoo," or "If you keep your room picked up, we will go play in the park." This approach would produce better results in maintaining a clean room than saying, "You have always been a messy child, and you will never change. You don't deserve to have fun."

Although you are no longer a little child, you still have a part of you that responds more favorably to kindness and acknowledgment than to criticism and reproach. Which way do you speak to yourself? The latter approach evokes resignation and disappointment, not motivation and commitment. And how we do one thing is how we do anything, so if you are stingy with yourself with celebration in weight-loss progress, you will also be in life and business ... and vice versa. Get the idea?

By the way, the Celebration, Acknowledgment, and Reward can be given to yourself from yourself, or you can request it from someone else as a support request. I often ask my husband, my coach, or another support person for acknowledgment when I can't access it for myself and my "not good enough" fear is at work.

Celebration can include rewards that cost nothing or that cost something. Either way, the important concept is the spirit of celebration, the spirit of acknowledgment, and the correlation or connection to the desired action or result.

By the way, when you are proactive in celebrating and acknowledging others, you also benefit. You practice seeing the world through the lenses of what's right, which flows over to you as well.

Even when we intellectually understand the concept of speeding up and empowering our results by practicing acknowledgment, celebration, and reward, many of us still don't do it. Many of my clients confuse the concept of what they already do, such as massage or buying clothes, with reward. Or they say they can't think of additional rewards; they already give themselves what they want. Correlation is the answer! Attaching the result or action to the reward involves your attitude about it.

If every week you enjoy a massage anyway, then it would not be correlated to your action or result. But if you now want to include it on your reward list, then you may correlate it any time you desire. For instance, when you drop the next five pounds, you will correlate that accomplishment with a 90-minute massage instead of 60 minutes. AND you further the celebration by telling the massage therapist that this is a special celebration to reward yourself for dropping five pounds. You have correlated the result with the reward.

Here is another example correlating your celebration. Let's say that you have had lunch with friends regularly, but now you want to include this lunch as your celebration for not having sugar for a week. So when you arrange the lunch, you tell your friend that you want to have lunch together to celebrate your accomplishment—a week of no sugar. At lunch you propose a toast (with water, tea, etc.) to yourself for accomplishing this goal. You have now correlated the result with the reward.

The correlation of the reward with the accomplishment is based on the spirit with which it is intended—not by rote or by mechanically going through the motions. Feeling joyful, exuberant, celebratory, and acknowledged are signs that you are giving yourself the spirit of celebration.

Gratitude

By practicing the attitude of gratitude, we allow ourselves to recognize ourselves and all the people, events, and experiences for which we are grateful. We see through the lenses of gifts, learning, and blessings. It's easier to be grateful for those things and people outside of ourselves, but not so easy sometimes to be grateful for qualities within ourselves. The same resistance described in the Celebration section applies to gratitude. In order to shift the Self-Deprecation pattern, an attitude of gratitude for ourselves, our abilities, and our qualities must be practiced, along with Celebration. It's the same deal: we focus on what's right, not on what's wrong with us.

I often give my clients a practice to look in the mirror each day and say, "I love and accept you just the way you are." I also ask them to notice what they are grateful for about themselves.

The following are ways to turn Self-Deprecation into gratitude:

- Instead of criticizing your fat stomach, be grateful for your body working well. When we are stressed or eat the wrong things, our bodies retain the fat as stored fuel. That's how it's supposed to work. Be grateful for that.
- Instead of criticizing your heavy thighs, be grateful for your strong legs that take you wherever you want to go.
- Instead of criticizing your inability to stick to a food plan, be grateful that we have so many food choices in this country.

The more you practice gratitude, the more at peace you will be with yourself and your world. The more peaceful you are, the more you will be in your Essence and will make your decisions regarding food, movement, and everything else from empowered commitment.

Service

Being of service and allowing yourself to be served provide an often overlooked opportunity to shift Self-Deprecation. When we are being of service or allowing ourselves to be served, the self-critical sabotage dissolves. We feel valuable and worthy when we are serving someone else. When we allow ourselves to be served, we are declaring ontologically that we are valuable and worthy too. The martyrdom and victim mentality shifts to self-love and self-worth. Service can be as small as asking someone to pass the salt or give you a back rub. It can be bigger, such as hiring a housekeeper or someone to prepare your tax return. Requesting service can include asking someone to listen to you or requesting support.

You may request service for yourself or offer service to another person. Both actions help you to shift the context of worthless, and therefore the sabotage of Self-Deprecation, to "I am valued and valuable." Do you of a certain age remember the mantra of Stuart Smalley on the *Saturday Night Live* television program? He looked at himself in the mirror while saying, "I'm good enough, I'm smart enough, and doggone it, people like me!" This was a comedy routine to spoof self-help strategies, but the meaning is valid. If we value and respect ourselves, we break out of the Self-Deprecation sabotage pattern that makes us feel bad and causes us to give up before we reach our goals. And we shift with practicing and asking for service.

Self-Deprecation slyly and surely degrades your abilities to keep your weight off. I suggest you consciously begin to notice self-deprecating thoughts or words and then substitute empowering, uplifting ones. You might begin with recording your big and small accomplishments in a journal every day. Combined with gratitude and service (for yourself and others), these habits will help you shift out of self-deprecation if done consistently.

Reason 9:
Suppression

Life is not about hiding and seeking, nor is it about learning the things you've forgotten
—no, it's not even about remembering them. It's about BEING! BEING YOURSELF!
You were Born to Expand the Infinite Nature of God. Live only to be who you are now. You are Creation's first and last hope to fill the shoes you alone can fashion, and eternity will pass before this chance will come again.
You are a dream of a legion before you who has passed on the torch of Space-Time awareness so that your mere existence could immeasurably enrich All That Is God.
By simply BEING, you will fulfill this dream, centered in the Here and Now, where all dreams come true, all truths reside, and understanding is born.
Your sacred heart was hewn at the dawn of creation in a dance to celebrate the birth of forever. You can do no wrong. There are no "should's," or "should not's," "rights," or "wrongs." Life is not about being happy, sad, good or bad. It's not even about making your dreams come true—that much is inevitable!
There is only BEING. Eternal BEING. Inescapable BEING. You are perfect. It is done.
Your rare and precious light has, and will forever more, illuminate the worlds you create ...
the worlds that now wait ... for your blessed BEING.
—Mike Dooley, *Lost in Space*

The Sabotage Pattern

*T*he sabotage pattern of Suppression is the result of self-deprecation and self-criticism. When we think we aren't good enough, we shut ourselves down ... or at least we don't fully express ourselves, and we don't play full-out in life. Our life purpose, as we discussed in sabotage #4, Playing Small, doesn't get realized or even lived in to. When we are not in alignment with who we really are and when we are not living our lives fully, we tend to stuff the unfulfilled needs with our compulsions—food, spending, drinking, inactivity, etc. Suppression takes Playing Small down even further because we put a barrel over our light.

Suppression has been taught to us from an early age. Did your parents teach you, "Children should be seen and not heard," or "If you can't say anything nice, don't say anything at all"? Did they teach you, "Don't speak unless spoken to" or "Big boys/girls don't cry"?

Even as adults we learn to suppress our feelings. When I was a Senior Sales Director for an international direct sales company, we were trained to respond to the question, "How are you?" with the answer, "Grrrrrreat!!!!" And if we were not really great, the answer was to be, "Unbelievable!" This was code for, "I'm NOT great, but it's not OK to talk about it." Never was there permission to say the truth if we were frustrated, disappointed, or unmotivated.

We have also learned early on that expressing emotions can be dangerous. Many of my clients, especially men, do not let themselves cry or otherwise show sadness or grief. They have been taught that it's a sign of weakness in our culture. Many of my clients, often women, do not let themselves show anger. They have been taught that it's selfish or unladylike. Some people believe that if they let their anger out, it will never stop and will become destructive, like an unleashed rabid tiger.

Suppression can include not only the "downside" emotions, but also the "upside" emotions. We have been taught that it's not okay to be too happy or too peaceful or too ecstatic, because something might happen to destroy it or we might offend someone else.

As a child I was very dramatic, both with my joyful dancing and singing at the top of my lungs and also with crying hysterically when I was upset. Time after time (on both ends of the emotional spectrum), my parents chastised me and demanded that I calm down.

Later in life, my husband advised me to "dial it down" with regard to expressing my opinions to his mother.

As in these examples, people are uncomfortable with our full range of expression, so we learn that we have to suppress it. People are also uncomfortable with their full magnificence and purpose.

Emotions, needs, dreams, and celebrations that are not "appropriate" to share get stuffed down with overeating or overdrinking. They may leak out in other ways, but the authentic, intentional expression is missing. And with our inner fears of "not good enough" or "not lovable," we try even harder to fit in to a definition of acceptable.

I have a friend who confided that she had accomplished the best year ever in her business. I was delighted for her and asked about the celebration party. She told me decidedly that she wasn't going to tell anyone else because people would be jealous or resentful. What?!!! She was suppressing herself to not make someone else uncomfortable.

Whenever I see someone who is overweight, I wonder what they would be like if they gave themselves permission to be the fabulous person they really are.

Suppression is also a sabotage pattern when we rebel against it. Teenagers who act out in various dramatic ways are reacting to suppression. The men in midlife crises with red sports cars and 18-year-old blondes are reacting to prior suppression in their lives.

In weight loss, Suppression can result in "stuffing," as mentioned previously, or in rebelling.

"Little Rebel" and "Ruby Rebel" are PDM names that I often give to clients who won't stick to their programs. They suppress their authentic selves in so many other ways that food and movement are the only means they know to express themselves and to "do whatever I please."

So the Suppression sabotage pattern leaks out in destructive ways when we don't give ourselves permission to be real.

What to Do About It: Authenticity, Full Expression, and Playing Full-Out

---

If you want to play the game of life and win,
you've got to play full out.
—Anthony Robbins

The shift from the sabotage pattern of Suppression is Authenticity—being your authentic self, which is your Essence. The shift also involves Full Self-Expression of that Authentic Self and Playing Full-Out in whatever you do in life. You could say that the shift comes from a willingness to live life instead of settling for a half-life.

"But that is risky!" you say to me. Yes, there are risks to Authenticity, Full Expression, and Playing Full-Out. You have to get out of your comfort zone of same old, same old. You have to be willing to be great. You have to own your gifts and talents in order to take them to the world. You have to give up caring what other people say and instead listen to your own heart. You have to give yourself a celebration party when you accomplish a goal. You have to accept your emotions. You have to summon the courage to get your needs met.

And there are benefits to Authenticity, Full Expression, and Playing Full-Out! You don't have to feel like a fraud. You don't have to hide your faults and hope no one discovers them. You don't have to work so hard to have people like you, because you now like yourself. You have a sense of freedom and aliveness. You get to experience life to its fullest without wishing, hoping, hiding, being stifled and afraid. You don't have to eat to stuff or rebel. You get to have energy, life, zest, and joy. You get to step out of fear and live life on purpose.

> *A life lived in fear ... is a life half-lived.*
> —Baz Luhrmann, *Strictly Ballroom*

And if you don't, well, you get to stay suppressed, which could be comfortable, safe, and easy. But it denies and disappears who you really are.

Making the Shift

How do we practice authenticity, full expression, and playing full-out? The first step is to declare that you are willing and able to do so. Then take action with a few practice suggestions, as follows:

- Acknowledge and celebrate your value, your gifts, and your talents.
- Realize you make a difference.
- Be yourself.
- Be fully present, undistracted by anything else.
- Stretch yourself, even if it makes you feel uncomfortable.
- Express yourself.
- Give it everything you've got—whatever the "it" is.
- Celebrate and acknowledge your big and small victories, as we discussed in shift #8.
- Notice when you bad-mouth (criticize) yourself. Rephrase the sentence to include what you did right.
- Practice celebration and acknowledgment of yourself and others for big and small victories as you did in shift #8.

- Notice when you suppress yourself in thoughts, actions, emotions, or dreams. Do the opposite, and deal with the consequences.
- Give your best effort, even if you want to quit.
- Make a decision to play full-out in all areas of your life. Decide what that looks like to you. Practice doing it.

What is the truth about yourself? Do you have the courage to practice speaking the truth about yourself, your emotions, and your needs? What's scary about expressing them? If you didn't gloss over them, what would that open up for you?

What would happen if you gave everything you do your full attention and energy? If you didn't hold back, went beyond what is comfortable, and played your game of life as if you didn't have a second chance, what benefit could emerge for you?

You've gotta dance like there's nobody watching,
Love like you'll never be hurt,
Sing like there's nobody listening,
And live like it's heaven on earth.
—Author unknown

Conclusion And Resources

*P*ermanent weight loss and maintenance involve a much deeper focus than food and exercise. When you learn the nine reasons you sabotage your success and when you begin to integrate new ways of empowering yourself, then your journey to forever fit, fat-free, and fabulous becomes successful and fulfilling. Ontological Weight Loss is indeed a Once-in-a-Lifetime Solution.

You don't have to do this alone! Some people need help beyond a self-help book, because they revert to old patterns. Whether you are a weight-loss coach or a weight-loss client, I am the perfect mentor to guide you to permanent weight-loss success. Here's how we can begin:

Sign up now for all three of the following free resources:

1. Download the "**Weight Loss 101 Package**" to help jump-start the journey to permanent weight loss. It includes several basics that every weight-loss professional and overweight person needs in their toolkit: Download your complimentary "Weight Loss 101 Package" at www.JanisPullen.com.

2. Schedule a complimentary "**Lose Weight for Life Consultation**" to discover ways in which you may continue working with Janis. Apply for your session at www.JanisPullen.com

3. Subscribe to weekly online **O.W.W.L. (Ontological Wealth, Weight, and Leadership) Success Tips** at www.JanisPullen.com

For additional information, please visit **www.JanisPullen.com**.

Appendix 1:
Weight And Health

When we think about overweight and obesity, we often consider the effects of weight on our lifestyle and well-being. We are impacted by lack of energy, lethargy, fatigue, discomfort, frustration, embarrassment, sex and intimacy worries, shopping inconvenience, time spent deciding what to wear, etc.

Most people also know that obesity contributes to physical breakdowns, such as heart disease and type 2 diabetes. Research shows that there are also many more correlations between weight and physical health, including gallstones, low energy, cancer, joint pain, and arthritis.

Excess weight also damages mental and emotional health, affecting self-worth, self-esteem, confidence, motivation, depression, anxiety, intimate relations, body image, weight discrimination, and joy of life.

In addition to the risks of obesity, excess sugar contributes significantly to many ailments of which we might be unaware. Excess consumption of sugar is linked to diabetes, arteriosclerosis, breast cancer, depression, foggy-headedness, nervousness, and osteoporosis—plus many other ailments.

For detailed lists of "Health Risks of Being Obese" and "Ailments Linked to Sugar Excess," please visit http://www.owlweightloss.com/weightloss101/ to request your free "**Weight Loss 101 Package**."

"I enrolled in the O.W.L. Coach Certification and Training Program because, as a holistic nutritionist, I am already offering the facilitative portion of weight loss (food and movement). I believe that the emotional side of weight loss is the most important part of the process.

"I found it very exciting to experience in my clients the transformations they made in their weight and also in other areas of their lives. Janis says, 'How you do weight is how you do everything!' These sabotage patterns really do work in every area of life: money, weight, health, relationships."

—Kristen Owens, Ontario, Canada. Holistic Nutritionist

"I hired Janis to be my life coach when my life had spiraled into a dead end. Over the course of a year, Janis worked with me to transform not only my personal life but also my professional career. I am a new woman—a confident, independent, and happy woman who has rediscovered her joy again. I'm deeply grateful to Janis for her patience, compassion, tenacity and professionalism. Please feel free to contact me regarding a recommendation for Janis."

—Gale O'Brien, Tijeras, NM. Author, Speaker, Cancer Survivor, and Wellness Advocate

Appendix 2:
Weight, Stress, And Money

*T*here is a surprising correlation between weight and money, which interests me greatly as a weight-loss expert and a money expert.

In addition to the health risks and ailments of being overweight, we incur financial risk as well, both as individuals and as organizations. Stress is the primary cause of physical and emotional disease, including heart disease, cancer, high blood pressure, inflammatory illnesses, anxiety, depression, and weight gain. And financial worries are among the top causes of stress.

There is a link between money and weight, with stress being the connection. Do you relate to any of these: stress eating, too much debt, not earning what you deserve or need, maybe earning plenty but not keeping enough of what you make? High stress provokes unhealthy emotional eating and overeating. But even if you eat reasonably well, chronic high stress results in weight gain. High stress, including financial stress, signals the body to produce cortisol, the fight-or-flight hormone, which physically tells the body to retain fuel (fat) in case of an impending emergency.

Interestingly, we experience stress when finances are strained, and we also experience stress when our wealth increases. So if our tendency is to engage in comfort eating or stress eating, we will gain weight when things are either bad or good. When a business fails or finances are in jeopardy, stress and weight can increase. When our income and responsibilities expand, stress and weight can increase. The common theme is stress.

Just as money affects weight, weight affects money. Statistics and observation show that there is a cost for being overweight, both in annual earnings and also in direct and indirect expenses.

The relationship between money, stress, health, and weight is so crucial that I have created a special program to help people create money breakthroughs and release financial stress. Many of my Weight of Money clients lose weight magically, and many of them enroll in the O.W.L. Weight Loss Program to continue their journey … and vice versa.

The following research findings reflect specific correlations between weight and money:

- Overweight women (those 25 pounds or more above normal weight) earn an annual average of $29,000 less than thin women.[13]
- Obese people are discriminated against when applying for jobs, are passed over for promotion, and are more likely to be made redundant—all purely on the basis of their weight.[14]
- Direct costs (such as medical expenses) and indirect expenses (such as lost wages and reduced work productivity) cost a man an average of an extra $2,646 annually if he is obese, and they cost a woman an average of $4,879 annually if she obese.[15]
- Employees' obesity-related health problems in the United States are costing companies billions of dollars each year in medical coverage and absenteeism. The nation's obesity rate has doubled in the last 30 years, and 34 percent of adult Americans are defined as obese. This contributes to a 36 percent increase in healthcare spending and five to seven percent of the national healthcare budget.[16]
- Experimental studies have found that when a résumé is accompanied by a picture or video of an overweight person (compared to an "average" weight person), the overweight applicant is rated more negatively and is less likely to be hired. Other research shows that overweight employees are ascribed multiple negative stereotypes, including being lazy, sloppy, less competent, lacking in self-discipline, disagreeable, less conscientious, and poor role models. In addition, overweight employees may suffer wage penalties, as they tend to be paid less for the same jobs, are more likely to have lower-paying jobs, and are less likely to get promoted than thin people with the same qualifications.[17]

- Overweight women are more likely to make less money than people of "normal" weight and, tellingly, plump women earn even less than men who are overweight or obese. A study by Jennifer Shinall, assistant professor of law at Vanderbilt Law School, showed that heavy women earned $9,000 less than their average-weight counterparts; very heavy women earned $19,000 less.[18]

The financial cost of obesity is clear. As we drop our excess weight permanently, we simultaneously drop other physical, emotional, and financial baggage.

"One of the most important results Ontological Weight Loss (O.W.L.) has produced for me in addition to weight loss has been an incredible confidence when it comes to my professional life. When I first started my business, I felt frumpy, and wanted to hide out where no one could see me because I felt so overweight. I hid behind my desk, behind my baggy clothes and by being quiet, not seeking the clients I knew I needed for my business to succeed. After entering O.W.L., I began to see how eating and weight gain were part of my hiding out as well. The holistic approach that Janis takes in the O.W.L. program affected not just weight, but my whole essence, and resulted in me feeling strong, confident, and owning my strengths and abilities—and that has meant a huge increase in clients and income. Thanks, Janis!"

—Debra Gilroy, PhD, East Springfield, PA. Psychologist

About The Author

I support extraordinary individuals and businesses
who are dedicated to creating incredible results and who
are willing to reinvent themselves in order to do so.
—Janis Charlton Pullen

Janis Pullen is an award-winning Executive Mastery Coach, Certified Money Breakthrough Coach, Master of Accountancy, retired CPA, and retired Senior Sales Director. She has taught hundreds of people to grow their businesses, achieve excellence, and flourish in life. Janis empowers and trains leaders to triumph in their physical and financial fitness, including weight, wealth, and leadership.

Releasing 50 pounds in the 1990s and being self-supporting for decades, Janis is passionate about helping people uncover their magnificence. She works with people who are committed to both personal and business success, including organizations, executives, and entrepreneurs who struggle with feeling stuck, stressed, overwhelmed, or overweight, so that they can clean up their money issues, leverage their time, and shed their financial or physical weight in order to have healthy, balanced, and abundant lives.

Janis created and coaches the *Weight of Money Breakthrough Programs*, the *O.W.L. Weight Loss Programs,* the *O.W.L. Weight Loss Coach Certification and Training Programs,* the *Keep It Off Club,* the *Wealth and Leadership Advanced Coach Training Program*, and various other private and group coaching programs. She is a speaker, trainer, and published author.

Janis' passions include ballroom and Latin dancing, which she often integrates in coaching workshops and retreats. She loves camping and hiking in the mountains with her husband, Jay, as well as bicycling and daily walking in her wooded neighborhood. Janis has taught countless people to water-ski behind her inboard/outboard ski boat, and once competed in the New Mexico state water-ski slalom competition, where she took third place.

Mission

My mission in life is to be at cause for a world at peace, one person at a time. I want to leave a legacy of empowering people to step into their magnificence and to create lives they love.

My mission for Ontological Wealth, Weight, and Leadership (O.W.W.L.) is to provide a once-in-a-lifetime program for people worldwide who have struggled and suffered with weight issues, so that they can live their lives with exponentially expanded joy, freedom, and peace.

I train coaches, health-minded companies, and weight-loss professionals worldwide in my unique Ontological Weight Loss (O.W.L.): Your Once-in-a-Lifetime Solution methodology, so that they may build highly successful businesses, grow themselves to be "ultimate" coaches, and teach clients to love and respect themselves while dropping weight permanently and living the life of their dreams.

Education and Certification

- Certified Mastery Coach, December 2013
- Certified Money Breakthrough Specialist, July 2012
- Certified Niche Breakthrough Coach, October 2011
- Certified Coach, International Association of Women Business Coaches, June 2011
- Mentor Coach and Leader-in-Training, Accomplishment Coaching, 2006–2008

- Certified Coach, Accomplishment Coaching, March 2006
- Certified Public Accountant: State of Texas 1984, State of New Mexico 2002
- Facilitator Training Program, Newton Learning Corporation, Fall 2001
- Visionary Leadership Program, Newton Learning Corporation, January 2000
- Master of Accountancy, New Mexico State University, June 1983
- Bachelor of Accountancy, New Mexico State University, June 1981
- Foreign Studies Program, Spanish language focus, Colorado Women's College

Testimonials

"I have been working with Janis since 2007, first as a life coach, which evolved into a business coach, and now as an Ontological Weight Loss Certified Coach. When I first started this journey of being an Ontological Weight Loss Coach, I had no idea what was in store for me and how it would impact my life and the lives of my clients—present and future. As I have gone through the training, it has challenged me and changed my life. I now realize the incredible benefits of the program and how amazingly it will work for anyone, regardless of their shape, size, and age—male or female—as long as they are committed to their health and well-being and are willing to work the program.

"I'm not just talking about weight issues. The results I have gleaned from working with Janis are the home of my dreams, attracting my ideal clients, writing and publishing my first book (with more to come), creating several successful businesses, manifesting over $85,000 in income this past year, and loving the skin I'm in. I love who I am.

"The results from working with Janis can be anything you imagine. It will show up as healthier relationships with yourself and others. You will have a more defined and clearer picture of your present, which will carry through to your future as you attract and create the body, lifestyle, career, income and financials of your dreams. You will have more self-confidence and self-worth in addition to more love, appreciation and acceptance of yourself as you learn how to celebrate you and what you bring to this planet."

—Jeaninne Grayson, CEO and Founder,
S.O.A.R. for Life and Ananda Yoga and More

"This is to recommend Janis Pullen. I have worked with her closely for the past several years. She is fun and funny. She is powerful and compassionate. She is wise and willing to listen. In short, she makes it easy to be in the audience. People can see themselves in Janis. They relate to her and are inspired by her. She is professional and warm, beautiful and approachable, and knows her stuff as a leader. You will not be disappointed when you work with Janis. She is an extraordinary human being. I am honored to know her. It has been my pleasure to receive both her support and guidance. She is a devastating combination of brilliance and heart. Please feel free to contact me with any questions."

—Hans Phillips, Santa Cruz, CA. CEO and Ontologist, Ontoco
Executive Performance Consulting

"I have known Janis for many years, and have participated in workshops that she has led as well as one-on-one coaching. Janis' approach to public speaking and workshops is straightforward, truthful, interesting, compassionate, humorous, prepared, and educated. She is a natural-born leader as well as speaker and conveyor of truth, inspiration, and information. One-on-one Janis exemplifies compassion, honesty, and confidentiality. The value I have received as a recipient of her coaching, as a workshop participant or audience member, is invaluable, important, and life-altering. Janis is a woman who walks her talk. I recommend Janis as a leader, speaker, or coach, and I am grateful for the opportunity to sing her praises. Please feel free to contact me for further information."

—Rita S. Stafford, Albuquerque, NM

Notes

1   "The Percentage of People Who Regain Weight After Rapid Weight Loss and the Risks of Doing So," Livestrong, last modified February 18, 2015, http://www.livestrong.com/article/438395-the-percentage-of-people-who-regain-weight-after-rapid-weight-loss-risks/.

2   "The 6 Human Needs: Why We Do What We Do," Anthony Robbins blog, August 7, 2013, http://training.tonyrobbins.com/the-6-human-needs-why-we-do-what-we-do/.

3   "Maslow's Hierarchy of Needs," Wikipedia, last modified February 18, 2015, http://en.wikipedia.org/wiki/Maslow%27s_hierarchy_of_needs.

4   "How Can I Use HALT to Fight Food Cravings?" Sharecare, accessed March 6, 2015, http://www.sharecare.com/health/nutrition-diet/how-use-halt-food-cravings.

5   "Ontological Weight Loss (O.W.L.): Your Once-in-a-Lifetime Solution," http://www.owlweightloss.com/programs/ontological-weight-loss-program/.

6   Mary O'Malley, *The Gift of Our Compulsions: A Revolutionary Approach to Self-Acceptance and Healing* (Novato, California: New World Library, 2004).

7   Star Trek database: Borg, accessed March 6, 2015, http://www.startrek.com/database_article/borg.

8   Audiobook (Nightingale-Conant, 1997). Available via Amazon at http://www.amazon.com/JOURNEY-THE-BOUNDLESS-Exploring-Connection/dp/0671577506.

9   Don Miguel Ruiz, *The Four Agreements: A Practical Guide to Personal Freedom*, ed. Janet Mills (San Rafael, California: Amber-Allen Publishing, 1997).

10   Susan Campbell, *Getting Real: Ten Truth Skills You Need to Live an Authentic Life* (Tiburion, California: H J Kramer/New World Library, 2001).

11   Marianne Williamson, *A Return to Love: Reflections on the Principles of "A Course in Miracles"* (New York: HarperCollins, 1992).

12   Eckhart Tolle, *A New Earth: Awakening to Your Life's Purpose* (New York: Penguin, 2008).

13   Freek Vermeulen, "The Price of Obesity: How your salary depends on your weight," *Forbes*, March 22, 2011, accessed March 6, 2015, http://www.forbes.com/sites/freekvermeulen/2011/03/22/the-price-of-obesity-how-your-salary-depends-on-your-weight/.
   Ashley Lutz, "This Chart Shows How Your Weight Affects Your Salary," *Business Insider*, April 11, 2012, accessed March 6, 2015, http://www.businessinsider.com/overweight-women-make-less-2012-4#ixzz2EEKAhsdG.
   Timothy A. Judge and Daniel M. Cable, "When it comes to pay, do the thin win? The effect of weight on pay for men and women," *Journal of Applied Psychology* Vol 96(1), Jan 2011, 95–112. http://dx.doi.org/10.1037/a0020860. (Paywall).

14   Juliette Kellow, BSc RD, "Fattist Employers Need to Work Things Out," Weight Loss Resources, accessed March 5, 2015, http://www.weightlossresources.co.uk/body_weight/obesity_discrimination.htm.

15   Tara Parker Pope, "Obesity More Expensive for Women," *New York Times*, September 27, 2010, accessed March 6, 2015, http://well.blogs.nytimes.com/2010/09/27/obesity-more-expensive-for-women/?_r=0.

16 Katherine Torres, "Obesity Costly for Employers," *EHS Today*, April 11, 2008, accessed March 6, 2015, http://ehstoday.com/safety/ehs_imp_79689.

17 "Obesity, Bias, and Stigmatization," Obesity Society, accessed March 5, 2015, http://www.obesity.org/resources-for/obesity-bias-and-stigmatization.htm.

18 Suzanne McGee, "For women, being 13 pounds overweight means losing $9,000 a year in salary," *The Guardian* US money blog, October 30, 2014, accessed March 6, 2015, http://www.theguardian.com/money/us-money-blog/2014/oct/30/women-pay-get-thin-study.

22474302R00085

Made in the USA
San Bernardino, CA
08 July 2015